THE POLITICS OF BREAST CANCER SCREENING

This book is dedicated to Peter, Jessica, Amy, Ben and the whole Faulkner family, who are too numerous to list individually. May you all live long and prosper!

The Politics of Breast Cancer Screening

ALISON HANN

Avebury

Aldershot • Brookfield USA • Hong Kong • Singapore • Sydney

Published by
Avebury
Ashgate Publishing Limited
Gower House
Croft Road
Aldershot
Hants GU11 3HR
England

Ashgate Publishing Company
Old Post Road
Brookfield
Vermont 05036
USA

British Library Cataloguing in Publication Data

Hann, Alison
     The politics of breast cancer screening –
     (Developments in Nursing and Health Care; no. 9)
     1. Breast – Cancer – Diagnosis – Political aspects
     2. Breast – Examination – Political aspects
     I. Title
     616.0'94'49

ISBN 1 85972 323 3

Library of Congress Catalog Card Number: 96-83267

Printed and bound by Athenaeum Press, Ltd.,
Gateshead, Tyne & Wear.

Contents

Acknowledgements

First of all, and most importantly, I must give my sincere thanks to my two long suffering supervisors. Professor Albert Weale and Dr John Street. If it had not been for Albert Weale, then I would never have had the confidence or the courage to start my thesis, let alone complete it. He has been a constant source of help, support and encouragement, and deserves a medal for patience in the face of sometimes unbelievable provocation! John Street had the misfortune to 'inherit' me when Professor Weale moved on, and consequently got the worst end of the deal because I was by this time fed up to the back teeth. He has also been incredibly supportive (if at times a bit picky) and he has helped me through a pretty diabolical couple of years. Thanks John, you probably don't realise what a great support you have been. I would also like to thank Jacquie White, who has guided me through the complexities of word processing. She has also helped me through panic attacks when I thought that I had accidentally erased all my files. Another source of encouragement has been Nick Everitt, whose constructive criticism has been incredibly helpful — I couldn't have got this far without him. I must also thank particular members of my family who have been especially supportive: in particular my children, who have had to put up with my crankiness during the seemingly interminable time it took to write this book, my Aunty Anne and my Uncle Arthur whose encouragement has kept me going, and my Mum and Dad, they helped the most because they knew I would do it, when I often doubted. I also owe a debt of gratitude to Colin of Texprep in Brackley, whose patience and expertise got the camera ready copy in shape for me, on time not once, but twice! And last, but not least I would like to thank my Mum, who spent many tedious hours proof reading the text and correcting spelling mistakes for me. Thanks Mum!

1 The background to Forrest

1 The scope of the problem

a The statistical picture

Breast cancer is by far the most common form of cancer among women in the U.K., currently accounting for 20% of all female cancer deaths and 4.5 per cent of the total number of female deaths. Figures from the, *Cancer Statistics Registrations*, published by the Office of Populations and Surveys suggests that the situation has been worsening slowly but steadily for a number of years. In 1971, the incidence of breast cancer was 18,182. By 1978, the figure had climbed to 21,486. From 1979, the statistics for incidence were compiled on a different basis, and breast cancer in situ was recorded separately from 'proper' breast cancer. Combining those two figures gives a figure for 1979 of 25,850; and since that year, the steady upward spiral has continued. In 1986 (the year in which the Forrest Report was published) the incidence was 37,416, and two years later, the figure topped 46,000.

Nor is merely the incidence of the disease which shows an alarming increase: the data also shows a steady annual increase, rising from 9,841 in 1964 to 13, 641 in 1986. The majority of breast cancers occur in older women, that is in women aged 60 years of age or over; but the incidence of the disease increases for all women beyond the age of 35. These figures showing national increases in incidence and death rates are part of a similar world-wide trend.

At present, the exact cause of breast cancer is not understood and there is no immediate prospect of primary prevention. Advances in treatment have achieved only modest increases in survival of women with symptomatic disease. Recent statistics concerning the national survival figures for England and Wales show a five year survival rate of 64 per cent, but the disease is still likely to recur for a period of at least twenty to twenty five years after diagnosis. It is thought that two thirds of women who develop breast cancer will eventually die from it. The survival rate is heavily dependent on the stage at which the cancer is discovered, and it is commonly thought in both medical and 'lay' circles that the earlier that a cancer is detected then the better are the chances of a recovery. In Britain, one of the main problems is that women tend not to present, even if they have discovered a lump, and even if they do so immediately, then the disease is often already at a fairly advanced stage. The problem of breast cancer is both a difficult one to solve and also a problem that effects a large number of women.

b Psychological impact for women

The threat of breast cancer is one that looms large in the female consciousness. Most women are aware that the disease is on the increase and that once diagnosed a woman faces at best disfiguring surgery, and at worse the loss of life. Increasingly, the setting up of the breast cancer screening service, and the controversy surrounding it (at whatever level) has been perhaps the single most important instrument which has made the threat of breast cancer more 'real', and yet in another way more vague. It has become more real

2

because women are generally more aware of the statistics concerning breast cancer incidence, and even if they do not know the exact figures, most are aware that it is a disease that can effect as many as one in eight women at some point in their lives (WHO, 1991). But it has also become more vague, inasmuch as there seem to be no clear-cut causes of cancer. There is evidence to suggest that certain factors which seem to increase the likelihood of developing the disease, such as age and social class (Forrest Report, 1986), but the links are relatively weak and uncertain. Breast cancer, then, can be perceived as a kind of unguided missile which can strike more or less at random.

Furthermore, exactly how the disease (once accurately diagnosed) is managed is highly dependent upon the region in which the woman happens to be resident, and on who her consultant surgeon is. Some surgeons favour radical surgery, while others do not. And which treatment women are likely to receive can therefore vary radically from one hospital to another, and may even vary within individual hospitals, depending on which surgeon treats the case. This variation reflects the lack of consensus within the medical profession over the most effective method of managing the disease.

c The role of the media in spreading awareness

It has also been a problem that has attracted an increasing amount of both public and medical attention. Articles concerning both breast cancer and breast cancer 'prevention' have been occurring regularly in women' magazines such as *Today, Cosmopolitan and Womans Own* for a number of years, and articles and features have appeared in the broadsheet 'quality' press such as the *Sunday Times* and *The Guardian* since the early 1970's. *The Sunday Times* for example (June 22nd and 29th 1980), ran a two week special on the problem of breast cancer, which showed how women could examine their breasts for lumps, and what the options for a woman were if she were unlucky enough to discover a lump. There have also been discussions in the press about the ways in which various well-known women, such as Nancy Regan (who underwent a mastectomy) have coped with the problem of breast cancer.

Unlike cervical cancer, breast cancer incidence is greater in women in the higher social classes, who form the main readership of the newspapers and magazines which were involved in the ongoing discussion over both the threat of breast cancer and the various forms of 'prevention'.

2 Activities of pressure groups

Concern over the increasing incidence of breast cancer in the US led in 1971 to the first large scale clinical trial of breast cancer screening using mammography, (Shapiro, 1991). This trail was to be the first of many, both in America and in Europe, which were concerned specifically with the effectiveness of screening for breast cancer by using periodic mammograms. The results of most of the trials seemed promising (although as we shall show later, this interpretation of the results is highly contestable — see chapter 2). As a consequence, by the late 1970s, pressure from various groups had begun for the government to set up a screening service for women at risk, or to initiate a trial of breast cancer screening in the UK (or both). This pressure continued to grow in the period between 1979 (when the first UK trial of breast cancer screening was announced), and the eventual decision to set up a nationwide breast cancer screening service in 1987. Some of these groups came from within the medical community. The Cancer Research Campaign, for example, found the results of the overseas tests so impressive that they felt that there was no need for further trials in the UK, and consequently urged the immediate setting up of a nationwide system of screening. They argued that such a trial would merely replicate the findings of all the other trials. Other individuals, however, notably Sir Patrick Forrest, argued that the clinical trial was essential before large amounts of public money were committed to a breast cancer screening programme. But though there were disagreements between individuals and groups concerning the exact timing for the introduction of breast cancer screening, in general there seemed to be very little serious disagreement over whether or not it was a good idea.

The period, then, between 1979 and 1987 witnessed a great deal of political activity from a variety of groups to encourage the government to provide a breast cancer screening service. In order to get a flavour of this activity we would like to focus for a moment on three of these groups which acted independently of the main medical lobby.

Unlike AIDS, where the sufferers themselves have been very active in the campaign for government and media attention, in the case of breast cancer, campaigning (such as it is) has been carried out predominantly from within the medical profession, and a limited number of pressure groups who have a particular interest in women's health. This has led to a situation (which is by no means unique) where 'women's wants' are being expressed in both the medical and

4

political arenas by a relatively small number of activists who may or may not have vested interests, and who may or may not be aware of the technical complexities surrounding the medical controversy.

a Trade Unions

Between 1968 and 1978 the TUC General Council, through the Social Health and Environmental Protection Committee had been actively promoting both cervical cancer screening and breast cancer screening. The TUC General Council's sub-committee on health promotion (the Social Health and Environmental Protection Committee) the body charged with investigating the issue of women's health and making recommendations. This Committee had a total of 69 members, but of the 69, only 20 or so were actively involved in the workings of the committee — they turned up to committee meetings, read proposals, etc. It was this smaller group which considered the benefits of the various methods of breast cancer screening. Their *initial* conclusion was that 'none of the techniques [are] foolproof', but that they were nevertheless had reached 'general agreement on the value of self-examination'. It is interesting to note that like many other lay groups and organisations, the TUC Subcommittee thus initially accepted, apparently without question, that breast self-examination is effective and valuable, which suggests that they were either unaware of the evidence that suggested that the practice was not useful, or they knew about it but decided to ignore it. Having spoken to someone who was a member of the Subcommittee at the time, We believe that the most likely hypothesis is that the members of the Subcommittee were unaware that the practice of breast self-examination was in any way controversial. This is perhaps an indicator of the depth (i.e. the shallowness!) of the investigation by the sub-committee. It is an important point to be borne in mind in considering their subsequent support for the screening programme.

Having thus initially favoured self-examination, the Subcommittee became aware of the rising number of deaths from breast cancer. In order to cope with this increasing problem, the Subcommittee at the 1981 General Congress launched a two-pronged attack. Firstly, and most importantly, the government should introduce a national breast cancer screening service, and secondly, action should be taken at the level of the workplace.

The 1981 TUC Congress Report took up both of these proposals. On the issue of a national screening programme, it reported that:

5

Partly as a consequence of TUC pressure, the previous government instituted a long term study of NHS breast cancer screening services (1981, pp. 38-60)

And on action the workplace level, the Report announced:

The emphasis is on action which unions could take at workplace level, and through collective bargaining to improve the health of women. It concentrates on the aims of expanding workplace health education projects for pregnant women: making it possible for every working woman to take advantage of services for breast cancer and cervical cancer screening . . . (1981, p. 57)

More specifically, the TUC General Council advised unions to undertake three initiatives to ensure that all women were screened for breast and cervical cancer: they should distribute to members, literature describing breast self-examination, and they should encourage women to take advantage of the services that were already functioning, and lastly, union officers should approach the Health Education Officer of the Local Health Authority to press for provision of free screening services in the workplace.

Between 1979 and 1987, the TUC passed a number of resolutions along these lines, both at the General Conferences and at the women's conferences, where the pressure on the Government was steadily growing, as was the frustration at the Government's inaction. The TUC, then. was one of the pressure groups (albeit not a very well-informed one) campaigning in favour of the provision of a national breast cancer screening programme.

b Women's National Commission

The Women's National Commission is an advisory committee to government whose remit is to ensure by all possible means that the 'informed opinions of women are given their due weight in the deliberations of government'. The origins of the commission lie in a body known as the Women Consultative Council which was set up in 1962 to keep the government of the day (Harold Macmillan's) 'in touch with women's thinking'. During the Wilson government, the Council was revamped and given more specific terms of reference. Today the Women's National Commission is a part of the Department of the Environment under the wing of Virginia Bottomley. It has 50 member organisations, and about 20 associate organisations. The current government co-chairperson is Baroness Denton, and her elected colleague is Mrs Margaret Morrison, former president of the civil service union.

In the November of 1984, the WNC published a report entitled *Women and the Health Service*. The report was concerned with a range of issues relating to women's health including cervical and breast cancer screening. Their methods of collecting information concerning 'women's thinking', at least as far as the 1984 report was concerned, were twofold. Firstly, a working group was formed by seventeen women. The Chairperson of the working group was Dame Alice Springman. She had been a member of the Social Science Research Council, and she had also been chairperson designate of the East Sussex Family Practitioner Committee. Of the other sixteen members of the committee, four members of the working group had a medical background. These were Professor Ruth Bowden who was a professor of anatomy at the University of London; Miss Catherine Caldwell, who was a senior midwife; Miss Margaret Lee who represented the Royal College of Nursing; and Mrs Joy Mostyn who was the regional administrator for the Family Planning Association, and who was also a member of the Women's National Cancer Campaign. The working group considered evidence from a wide range of experts covering a wide range of women's health issues. Of the 20 or so visiting experts, only one, Mrs Alice Burns, had any specialist knowledge concerning breast cancer screening. Mrs Burns had worked with the National Cancer Control Campaign studying the provision of screening services by the NHS.

On reading the proceedings we conclude that the information provided by the expert witnesses was accepted somewhat uncritically, and there is little to suggest from the report that the possible counter-arguments to the desirability of breast cancer screening were considered at all.

The other source of the WNC's information concerning 'women's thinking' was via public opinion:

> Comments were invited from both members of the public, and the Association of Community Health Councils for England and Wales. Various District Health Authorities and Scottish Health Boards were individually asked to comment on various aspects of their services (1984, p. 4)

The WNC also sent out questionnaires. The report mentions that they received 6,000 questionnaires back, but does not say how many were initially sent out, nor who they were sent to or how the sample population were chosen. In any case, the questionnaire did not contain any questions which related directly either to breast cancer or cervical screening .

In the light of their collected information the rather muddled report concluded that:

> Early detection [of breast cancer] greatly lessens the chance of the disease becoming fatal (1984, p. 20)

And the recommendation of the WNC was therefore that:

> Every woman is encouraged to develop the habit of self-examination of her breasts [and that] the current DHSS research into the effectiveness of mammography, clinical examination and education in self-examination for the early diagnosis of breast cancer are quickly utilised and published. (1984, p. 21)

Subsequently, however, the WNC added its voice to those campaigning in favour of breast screening by mammography.

c Royal College of Nursing

The Royal College of Nursing has a number of small bodies within it which focus on various specialist areas. One of these is the Breast Care Nursing Society. This group was formed by Mrs Sylvia Denton, and was initially called the Breast Care Forum. Throughout the period between 1979 and 1986 this group was extremely active in the promotion of breast cancer screening. Speaking of this period in an interview with me, Sylvia Denton remarked that:

> We believed passionately in breast cancer screening and were determined to keep the matter on the boil. We (the Breast Care Nursing Society) had regular press conferences at the Royal College, we lobbied Ministers, and we were constantly writing letters to magazines, journals and newspapers (1993)

Sylvia Denton focused her attention on the need for more and better trained nurses to help run an effective breast cancer screening service. Convinced (along with other members of the group) that a constant stream of media attention was essential to the cause of breast cancer screening, she was a tireless letter-writer, both to MPs and to the press. The group successfully lobbied Mrs Edwina Currie, (then a

8

backbench MP), who then became a supporter both of the increased training for nurses to help care for breast cancer patients, and also of the proposed breast cancer screening service. It was also partly due to the influence of the Breast Care Nursing Society (according to them) that Edwina Currie became interested enough in 1986 to travel to Sweden to see how they were running their breast cancer screening service, and for her to express publicly her support for the group to the media.

But Edwina Currie was not the only member of parliament to become involved with the group's activities. Mr Michael Hancock, who at the time was the Member of Parliament for Portsmouth South, had long been interested in health care policy, partly due to the influence of the Breast Care Nursing Society (again, according to them), and partly due to a close personal friend dying of breast cancer. He was very active in his own constituency, raising money for breast cancer screening equipment for use in Portsmouth South. During the course of 1986 he tabled two Early Day Motions in the House of Commons urging the government to adopt a breast cancer screening service.

As well as the three groups highlighted here as the most influential and well-organised, there were a number of other parties who were pressing for government action on breast cancer screening. But the mere fact that these groups were involved in involved in applying pressure does not mean that they were well-informed in the sense of being fully aware of the medical controversy surrounding mammography as a screening modality. Indeed, we have seen how in the case of the TUC Subcommittee, the opposite is the case. Rather, it seems that the Subcommittee, in common with some of the other groups involved, were not concerned with the details of the medical debate at all, but saw breast cancer screening as something which *must* of benefit to women, and so were anxious to exert pressure on that basis alone, without reference to 'real' medical evidence of benefit.

When it was announced that the Government were finally going to implement the recommendations of the Forrest Committee, most of the criticisms were not focused at all on the question of the efficacy of breast screening as a medical procedure. Rather, they were concerned with the question of whether the proposed level of funding was adequate, and of why the Government had not responded sooner to the recommendations made by the working group's interim report. For example, Michael Meacher asked in the House of Commons if the Secretary of State was aware that:

9

This was a grossly inadequate response to the Forrest Report, when 5,000 women had died of breast cancer while the government had been sitting on the report since last year? The six million announced today would not even fund screening for all women over 50. (Hansard, 1987)

In other words, the members of the House of Commons were not at all against the idea of a breast cancer screening programme — in fact, just the opposite. The objections were along the lines of 'too little too late'.

Outside the House, some criticisms of a different kind were voiced, although these again did not focus on the efficacy of breast cancer screening as such. Rather, the worry was about the cost of the service to the NHS. For example, the medical correspondent reported on July 19th in *The Times* that:

At present there seems little prospect of mass screening being offered by the Health Service to all women, even those over the age of 50. Use of the simplest screening methods seems unlikely to bring the cost below £50 for each women screened. (1987)

A similar worry was expressed in another article in *The Times* seven years later on September 14th, when Nicholas Timmins produced an estimate of the cost of finding a single case of breast cancer:

On this basis, it costs £80,000 to detect a single case of breast cancer because the chances of a case being discovered are one in five hundred. (1993)

We can thus see that there seemed to be a fairly solid consensus about the desirability of the breast screening programme. Pressure groups who could be expected to have women's health as a prime concern were in favour of it; high-profile women like Edwina Currie supported it; the House of Commons backed it; and the vast majority of the articles and newspaper stories at this time about the programme concentrated on the potential benefits. Thus the popular press presented a picture of an unproblematic screening service which could save hundreds (or thousands) of women's lives. What criticisms there were focused not on the utility of breast cancer screening as an effective medical procedure, but rather on practical question about the proposed mode of implementation by the Government, arguing either that the Government was being too niggardly, or alternatively that the Government proposals would too costly. It is thus unsurprising that it was assumed by the majority of the lay public that there was a high degree of consensus among the medical community concerning the usefulness of a national breast cancer screening programme.

We will show in Chapter 2 that this appearance of an informed consensus was misleading. But before revealing the details of the medical controversy surrounding breast cancer screening as such, we will sketch the Government's response to the pressure outlined above.

3 The response of the Government

a The pre-Forrest response

We have seen above in section (2) how by the late 1970s pressure was growing from various quarters for the government to set up a screening service for women at risk, or to initiate a trial of breast cancer screening in the UK (or both). On September the 4th 1978, David Ennals, the then Secretary of State for Social Services, announced that the Department of Health would be setting up a controlled trial. He said that if the results were favourable, then that might pave the way for a national breast cancer service. The UK clinical trial was to take seven years to complete. This trial, which actually began in 1979, was designed to examine and compare the effects of several different methods of detecting early breast cancer. These methods included mammography, breast self-examination (BSE), and clinical breast examination (CBE). The committee which was formed to run the trial was composed of 41 members, 15 of whom were later involved with the Forrest Committee, serving either as members or as consulting experts.

The initiation of the national trial was widely considered to be a major step towards the setting up of a UK breast cancer screening programme, as most people (both within medical circles and outside it) presumed that the UK trial would replicate the findings of the overseas studies which were claiming (on average) a 30% reduction in mortality rates from breast cancer.

b Setting up the Forrest Committee

In 1985, the Government finally announced that it was creating a

11

Working Party to look into the feasibility of breast cancer screening using mammography. They appointed as Chairman Sir Patrick Forrest, a leading expert in the field, who had already been active in setting up and participating in the 1979 committee referred to above which was running the national trials.

i The composition of the Committee

In addition to Forrest himself, there were a further eight members of the Committee, all of whom were picked by Forrest. There were also ten official observers, and a further 40 participating experts from a wide range of institutions and disciplines. (A full list of the members with brief biographical details is included in Appendix 2)

The setting up and composition of the Committee display several features which are particularly significant for our purposes. First is the selection of Forrest himself to head the Committee. He was of course already established as an expert in the field. But significantly, he was someone who had already committed himself to the desirability of setting up a national screening programme.

Secondly, there is the fact that all the remaining members of the Committee were picked by Forrest himself. None of them was a declared critic of a screening programme, and several of them were already declared supporters. Again, this is a significant fact. Given that the aim of the Committee was *not* merely to determine how to implement a programme that had already been decided to be valuable, but rather to determine whether or not it was valuable in the first place, one might have thought that to achieve balance, some known opponents of the programme would have been obvious appointees. There were, after all, some distinguished experts (such as Dr Petr Skrabanek and Dr Maureen Roberts) who were known beforehand to be critical of the idea of instituting a national screening programme. That it was thought right to include known supporters, while excluding known opponents, of the screening programme must make us think that the subsequent unanimous support of the programme by the Committee is less than surprising.

Thirdly, the sexual balance of the Committee is significant: of the nine members, only three were women. The reason that this is important is that the Committee were dealing with a disease which affects only women, and which both in itself and in the standard surgical response to it is *psychologically* traumatising for women. It is not unreasonable to think that although being male would not affect *some* areas of relevant expertise in discussing the disease (e.g. the assessment of statistical information, or the financial costing of different forms of treatment), it would be a major handicap in other relevant areas (e.g. in assessing the psychological impact on a woman of various kinds of medical procedure). It is worth noting that the only member of the Committee subsequently to have expressed reservations about the wisdom of the national screening programme which the Committee recommended was one of the women members, Dr Ruth Ellman (1989).

The suggestion is not of course that Forrest's earlier commitment to the screening programme led him to behave in any way improperly. The point is rather that given that the Committee was instructed to investigate the comparative merits of different methods of detecting breast cancer, it is not surprising that it came down in favour of mammography, given that it was chaired by someone who was already in favour, given that the other members of the Committee were chosen by that person, given that several of those other members were (like the Chair) antecedently committed to the desirability of screening, and given that none of the other members included any of the known opponents of mammography. These facts about the selection and prior commitments of members of the Committee certainly need to be borne in mind when we ask ourselves how far the Forrest Report can be regard as an impartial document produced by disinterested experts; and we shall accordingly be returning to this point in Chapter 3 and again in Chapter 5.

ii The terms of reference of the Committee

The Committee's terms of reference were:

> 1 To consider the information available on breast cancer screening by mammography: the extent to which this suggests necessary changes in the UK policy on the provision of mammographic facilities and the screening of symptomless women, (Forrest Report, p. 7) and

> 2 To suggest a range of policy options and assess the benefits and costs associated with them, and set out the service and planning manpower, financial and other implications of implementing such options. (Forrest Report, p. 7)

It is important to notice that there was nothing in these terms of reference which forced the Committee to take for granted that the

13

cancer screening programme was the only effective way of treating the problem: they would have been entirely within their terms of reference had they declined to go along with the consensus in public opinion noted in (2) above. They could have recommended delaying any decision until the result of the tests initiated in 1979 (referred to in (3) (a) above). The results were, after all, due two years months after the Committee published its Report. This availability of alternative recommendations which would have been fully within the Committee's terms of reference is a point to which we shall return in Chapter 3.

4 The workings/meetings of the Committee

The Committee met on eleven occasions, and read about 70 papers. Some but not all of the meetings were attended by the consulting experts, who were able to present evidence to the Committee. (Forrest, 1990). Unfortunately, no documentary records now remain of those meetings, and of the discussions which led to the Committee's recommendations: the minutes of the meetings have all been shredded. Furthermore, it has proved impossible to obtain any first-hand evidence about the meetings from members of the Committee. Sir Patrick himself has long been out of the country and unobtainable. The other members of the Committee, while not formally declining to be interviewed , have always in practice been unavailable for comment.

Evidence about the detailed workings of the Committee therefore has had to be gleaned (a) from the Reports issued by the Committee, and (b) from interviews with some of the consulting experts, such as Dr Skrabanek. But this has necessarily left blank a number of issues of interests, such as what proposals the Committee considered; what evidence for and against those proposals was examined, and what evidence was ignored; on what points there was disagreements within the Committee and on what points consensus, etc.

5 The recommendations of the Committee (The Forrest Report)

An Interim Report was published in January 1986 and reported that:

> The information that is already available from the principal overseas studies demonstrates that screening by mammography can lead to the prolongation of the lives of women aged 50 and over with breast cancer. There is a convincing case, on clinical

grounds, for a change of UK policy on the provision of mammographic facilities and the screening of symptomless women (p. 7)

The final Report, published later the same year, is fully in accord with the Interim Report. The committee believed that all the evidence was in favour of setting up a national breast cancer service, and that the benefits would far outweigh the costs. A member of the Forrest Committee remarked to me that after the publication of the interim report in January 1986, there was an air of expectation as the working group waited for the government to do something more definite about a national breast cancer screening service. It had been assumed that the interim report would initiate immediate government action.

The final Report was very detailed and made a range of recommendations. A summary of these are given in Appendix 1, but the principal recommendations were as follows:

1 Breast cancer screening with mammography should be implemented on a nation-wide basis for the screening of symptomless women (or at least those aged between 50 and 64).
2 Pilot centres should be set up to monitor and confirm the findings of the working group. (The committee fully expected the UK trial, (which was due to publish its findings in 1988) would replicate the findings of other favourable overseas trials — for details of these other trials, see Chapter 2)
3 High quality single medio-lateral oblique view mammography 'is the preferred basic screening method for mass population screening'.
4 Until the optimum frequency was determined, there should be an interval of three years between screening rounds.
5 An organisational structure should be set up to implement the findings of the committee.

6 The Government's response to the Report

To the surprise of the Committee, the Government did not respond at once to the interim Report, and there was some speculation that the costs involved in setting up and running the sort of scheme that the Committee favoured was meeting with Governmental opposition. However, in February 1987, a year after the publication of the interim report, (and incidentally three months before a general election), the

Secretary of State for Social Services, Norman Fowler announced the Government's intention to implement the Report:

> The Government accepts the proposals made in the report and accordingly have decided to implement a national breast cancer screening service. This will provide screening every three years for all women aged between 50 and 64 throughout the United Kingdom . . . We are determined that breast cancer screening should be implemented as effectively and as quickly as possible. We have therefore decided to provide additional funds for each Regional Health Authority to have at least one centre in operation within the next twelve months. (Hansard, 1987)

The allocation of earmarked money by the government may have been influenced by the problems encountered by the cervical cancer screening service which had tried to function without earmarked funds. For breast cancer screening, each Regional Health Authority was allocated £3,356,000 which included £150,000 for capital expenditure on buildings and equipment. (Forrest Report, p. 63) There was also a recurrent revenue allocation of £206,000 which was intended to meet the cost of setting up the screening centre and operating the call and recall system. These figures were for one 'Forrest' or one population.

The breast cancer screening service was to be organised through the Regional Health Authorities. Each screening centre was to serve a minimum population rather than a geographical area (such as a District Health Authority). The recommended size of the population was to be about half a million, which was roughly the population of two or three average sized District Health Authorities. Although the major organisational responsibilities for the programme were to fall to the Regional Health Authorities, in order for the service to run efficiently it was essential that there was a high degree of cooperation between the RHA and the Family Practitioner Committee (as it was then), consultants and GPs. The structure of the organisation was therefore as follows:

> *Department of Health* Defines aims and objectives of BCSP, allocates funds.
> *Regional Health Authority* Oversees management of screening centres nominates person responsible for BCSP, produces formal guidelines for QA for Region.
> *District Health Authority* Monitor women through the system,

collate data, budget holder and centre manager appointed.
General Practitioners Operate the call and recall system

The organisation of the system was designed to avoid many of the problems associated with the cervical cancer screening programme, which had attracted a great deal of media attention.

7 The 'commonsense' explanation of this series of events

The events described in this chapter thus seem to reveal a more-or-less rational sequence. A problem is identified; increasing public pressure forces the government to set up a committee, whose members are dispassionate professionals, who are highly regarded in their own fields. The committee is charged with producing the best form of medical care for a certain class of women, and accordingly the committee consults all the relevant research publications, and calls upon a wide range of other experts to submit expert testimony. A Report is produced which embodies their collective wisdom, and a screening programme is consequently set up. Our contention, by contrast, is that this interpretation of events is naive and simplistic, and that a better one can be found. We shall start the defence of the first part of this claim in the next chapter, by arguing that, even on the basis of the medical evidence which was available to the Committee, their own recommendations were importantly flawed.

References

Baker, J. (1982), 'Breast Cancer Demonstration Project: Five year Preliminary Report', *Cancer*, Vol 137, pp. 194-224.
Fagenberg, C, J, G., Tabar, L. (1991), 'Results of Periodic One-view Mammography Screening in a Randomised Controlled Trial in Sweden', *Screening For Breast Cancer*, Day and Miller (eds) Huber Publishers, Toronto Canada.
Forrest, A, P. (1986), 'Breast Cancer Screening: A Report to the Health Ministers of England and Wales', HMSO.
Forrest, A.P. (1990), *Breast Cancer: The Decision to Screen*, Nuffield Provincial Hospitals Trust, London.
Parliamentary Debates, (1987), *Hansard*, Sept 4th.
Report of the TUC Congress, 1981.

Shapiro, Venet and Strax, (1991), 'Current Results of Breast Cancer Screening Randomised Trials: The Health Insurance Plan (HIP) of Greater New York Study', *Screening in Health Care*, Walter Holland and Susie Stuart (eds), The Nuffield Hospitals Provincial Trust.

Timmins, N., (1987), 'Breast Cancer Screening', *The Times*, 19th July.

Verbeek, A., Hendricks,J., et al., (1984), 'Reduction in Breast Cancer Mortality Through Mass Screening with Modern Mammography: The First Results of the Nijimegen Project'. *The Lancet*, pp. 1222-4.

Women's National Commission, (1984), *Women and the Health Service*, Cabinet Office, WNC084/4.

2 The medical background to breast cancer

1 Medical details of cancer

Typically, invasive breast cancer forms a mass of tumour tissue in the breast that is hard and irregular and is integrated into the surrounding tissue. It often distorts the breast, and is often first noticed by a flattening of the normal smooth contour of the breast when the tissue is stretched by the woman raising her arms. Later though there is a more obvious asymmetry between the breasts. Distortion and contraction of the supporting tissues lead to the tethering of the skin over the tumour, and that of the ducts to an asymmetrical retraction of the nipple. If the cancer is superficially placed, then the skin becomes adherent to it and cannot be moved freely over the breast mass. If it is deep within the breast tissue, then it may become attached to the fascia that overlies the pectoral muscles themselves, and this also interferes with the free movement of the breast over the chest wall. The lymph nodes[1] in the axilla may become palpably enlarged. If a fine needle aspiration[2] is carried out, cancer is most commonly hard and gritty and the aspirate contains clumps of malignant cells. If the cancer is not diagnosed at this stage, then the tumour will continue to grow in size and may invade the skin forming a plaque of firm tumour tissue that may ulcerate. Invasion of the lymphatics in the skin gives rise to skin oedema[3] and the satellite nodules, invasion of the skin capillaries gives rise to a redness and swelling — the so called 'inflammatory cancer'. Should the tumour extend deeply to penetrate the muscle, it can become fixed to the chest wall and may even cause erosion of the ribs. The lymph nodes in the axilla become larger and, owing to the extension of the tumour the tissues become attached to one another, and to surrounding structures. At this stage, the lymph nodes in the neck can become involved and also the internal mammary nodes. But for most patients, it is not the local disease that is most feared, but the systemic spread of the disease. Common sites for secondary metastases[4] are the bone marrow, lungs, liver, brain and the pleural and peritoneal cavities; but no site is exempt. In 1953, the Union Internationale Contre Cancre introduced and international system for classifying breast and other cancers. This was based on a system developed by Pierre Denoix in France. The TNM system is now

[1] Lymph nodes are small accumulations of normal glandular tissue where lymphocytes are formed (lymphocytes are white blood cells involved in the immune system and in the combat of infection). In breast cancer, the condition of the local lymph nodes (in the axilla or armpit) is used to determine whether the disease has spread beyond the breast.

[2] Fine needle aspiration is a technique used to differentiate cysts from solid lesions in the breast. A needle is inserted into the lesion (or lump) and material is drawn out using a syringe. It can then be stained and the cells examined in a laboratory to find out whether the cells are benign or malignant.

[3] Oedema is an accumulation of tissue fluid in the tissues.

[4] Metastases are secondary cancerous deposits which have detached themselves from the primary tumour and established themselves to other sites.

accepted throughout the world as a standard measurement of the stage the cancer has reached. TNM stands for Tumour, Nodes and Metastases, each of which is classified according to the extent of involvement of the neighbouring tissues: N defines whether axillary and other regional lymph nodes are infiltrated by metastases or not; and M whether distant metastases are present or not. From TNM categories the stage of the disease is determined. In general, stage I disease is a small tumour limited to the breast; stage II is either a tumour of greater size or one associated with axillary node involvement. Stage III denotes locally advanced disease involving the skin or chest wall, and stage IV is the stage at which the disease is clinically shown to have moved to sites outside the local area. The influence of the stage at which the tumour is discovered and the prognosis for the women concerned can be seen in figure one.

2 Traditional methods of treatment

The surgical treatment for breast cancer became a standard part of the medical repertoire late in the last century. Prior to the introduction of anaesthesia and of antisepsis, only operations of absolute necessity were attempted. These involved the removal of ulcerating breast tissue. There was no expectation of cure. But with the development of painless, and relatively safe surgery, operations could be designed on anatomical and pathological principles and have clear objectives. For breast cancer these aims were the eradication of the visible tumour in both the breast and in the axilla.

The first such 'radical' operation was probably performed by Lister in Glasgow, just two months after he had used his carbolic treatment for a clean surgical wound. The patient was his sister, Isabella Pimm. She recovered well from the operation, and survived for three years without complications, when she died from a tumour of the liver (Forrest, 1989). Similar operations were soon being performed by other surgeons throughout europe. But relapse was very common, probably due to the fact that by the time the operations were performed the disease had already reached a very advanced stage. This high rate of relapse prompted Halstead to design the operation that came to be known as the Halstead radical mastectomy. His operation removed the breast and the underlying muscle clothing the rib cage, the pectorals. It also completely removed the lymph nodes in the axilla. Halstead's main objective was to achieve local control of the disease, and he mistakenly believed that he had found a cure for the disease. He wrote:

> If three years had passed without detecting either local recurrence or symptoms of internal disease, one could feel sure that a cure had been achieved (Halstead, 1907, p. 18)

The belief that this method of dealing with the disease was the only correct one was consolidated by Sampson Handley, who claimed that cancer spread through the body by a wavelike permeation of columns of cells along the lymphatic pathways towards the regional lymph nodes. Only when these nodes were breached did secondary disease develop. This erroneous belief, coupled with suggestions arising from Vichrows' work (1973) that the lymph nodes acted as a kind of filtering mechanism which filtered out embolised cells, established the idea that breast cancer was a regional disease, which was best cured by radical local therapy. The scope of radical surgery was therefore expanded into super-radical operations which removed the lymph nodes in the neck and from within the chest cavity, and even amputating the whole forequarter, and by introducing radical post operative radiotherapy to 'sterilise' the region of any residual cancer cells.

It took almost a century to prove that both the theory and the practice were wrong, firstly by experimental evidence, and secondly by results of a large number of randomised controlled trials which indicated that such 'heroic' methods of management did not improve the long term rate of 'cure'.

Not all surgeons however, had accepted the logic of radical surgery. In London, Patey doubted the necessity of sectioning the pectorals, and in his 'modified radical mastectomy' removed only the mammary gland and the lymph nodes in the axilla. In Edinburgh, McWhirter believed that it was illogical to treat the axillary nodes surgically and other nodal areas with irradiation, and he therefore advised surgeons to limit their operation to a removal of the breast alone (the so-called simple mastectomy), which then allowed the irradiation of the 'primary field' of lymphatic spread en block. Another surgeon, Keynes, suggested that radical surgery was both illogical and mutilating. He maintained that what was needed was systemic rather than local radical treatment. Others followed his example and abandoned radical surgery.

During this period of change, advances were being made in other areas of research concerning the morbidity associated with mastectomies. Tiona Morris, Greer and Maguire (1977) produced work which indicated that following mastectomy one in five women develop anxiety and depression of a moderate to severe degree (Morris, 1977; MacGuire, 1978). Patients had difficulty sleeping, and in dealing with every day problems, some were even afraid to leave their homes on their own. They lost interest in their homes and families, they ate badly and lost their sexual desire. It was initially believed that these effects were due to the loss of the breast, and there is no doubt that a mastectomy has its own psychosexual morbidity. But it is not just the mastectomy which causes morbidity of this type. There seem to be other factors at work, including the fear of the disease, lack of confidence in their doctor, and guilt that perhaps a faulty personality or a faulty life-style had caused the cancer.

Given, therefore all of the problems associated with the surgical management of the disease there was considerable pressure to find less invasive (and more effective) methods of dealing with the disease.

As invasive cancer is potentially a systemic disease, one such method of controlling the disease might be found in the effective treatment for micro-metastatic spread. An early method of achieving this was the removal of the ovaries, which was introduced in 1895 by Sir George Beatson. He observed evidence of a relationship between the ovarian hormones, oestrogen and progesterone and cancer of the breast. (Early Breast Cancer Trials Group, 1985). It was recognised that the beneficial effects of oophorectomy (the removal of the ovaries) on advanced disease was limited to pre-menopausal women, but this observation led later to the removal of the adrenal gland, and also to the removal or the destruction of the pituitary gland. (It is now known that the effect of this operation is to deprive the tumour of oestrogen).

During this period of endocrine surgery, pharmacological agents which were capable of antagonising the effects of oestrogen were also being used for the relief of advanced disease. Such agents were largely reserved largely for the management of life threatening conditions, and were not given with any hope or expectation of cure. Indeed, although some effect of these measures had been noted, the benefits to the patient of such measures, in terms of their improved survival or quality of life seemed negligible. A similar problem existed with the use of surgery: however radical the operation might be, the chances of survival for five years or more after the treatment were very slim.

However, there was some evidence to suggest that systemic therapy for early disease might be possible. This evidence came from a series of controlled trials in which systemic treatment has been given as adjuvant therapy. The first such trial was of suppression of ovarian function by radiation in 1953. Later studies concentrated on the effects of tamoxifen and of chemotherapy; and there now appears to be unequivocal evidence that both give benefits. This comes from the report of the Early Breast Cancer Trials Co-operative group, which under the leadership of Richard Peto in Oxford, carried out an overview analysis of the mortality results of all randomised trials world-wide of adjuvant tamoxifen and chemotherapy; these trials together included over 30,000 women. (Early Breast Cancer Trials Group, 1985). There were 28 trials of tamoxifen including 16,000 women, and its administration over a period of two years led to a significant reduction in mortality.

It is thus apparent that traditional treatment for cancer was unsatisfactory. The disease was diagnosed late in its development, the treatment involved major surgery, the patient was left traumatised, and the success rate was poor. Clearly, then, there was a need for some alternative approach.

3 Methods of diagnosis

Traditional methods of treatment relied on a diagnosis which was imitated by the woman herself. She would discover lumps in the breast by chance (in fact, the lumps were often discovered by the woman's partner), contact her doctor, and a diagnosis would then be made, often followed by surgery. Approximately 90% of reported breast lumps were first identified in this way. The problem with this approach is that by the time the lump was large enough for the woman to notice it, and for her to present, the cancer would be as a fairly advanced stage, and the prognosis would poor.

What was needed, therefore, was a method of identifying the tumours early. This would have two advantages: first, the tumour could be removed before dissemination had occurred, and thus the need for major and psychologically disturbing surgery such as mastectomy would be removed. Secondly, and as a consequence of the first, the prospects of a cure would be improved.

It was with this need for early diagnosis in mind that an educational programme was initiated by Community Health Councils, Family Planning Clinics and GPs. The aim of the programme was to teach women how to examine their breasts regularly and in an informed way for very small lumps. Although the appeal of this approach is clear from what has been said above about the inefficacy of relying on chance discover of breast lumps, it is nonetheless surprising that breast self-examination (BSE) as it was called, should have gained the backing medical bodies. For there was already evidence from clinical trials suggesting that BSE was ineffective (Day and Miller, 1987; Hill, 1988; Hobbs, 1985, Dixon, 1987).

4 Screening with mammography

There was, however, an alternative to BSE: breast cancer screening by mammography. As the details of this procedure will important in the overall argument of the thesis, this method will be described in some detail.

Its origins lay in the late nineteenth century. Following the discovery of x-ray imaging in 1895 by Roentagen, a German pathologist, Salomon, used the technique to examine the breasts of women who had died of breast cancer, so that he might study the pattern of malignancies within the breast tissue. He found that malignant clumps of cells (some of which were too small to be felt), appeared on the mammogram as small black spots. These micro-calcifications were not detectable using any other method, and Solomon realised that the mammogram might therefore be a way of detecting occult cancer of the breast. Following the first world war, there were attempts to use the mammogram to examine the breasts of living patients. But it was to be decade before the technology was developed which would allow pictures of a living breast which were detailed enough accurately to detect micro-calcifications. By the late 1970s, machines had been developed which provided very good 'views', and many radiography departments were using mammograms as a diagnostic tool for women with symptomatic breast disease.

What a universal programme of screening by mammography involves is that *every* woman, whether antecedently displaying any symptoms or not, is invited for a mammographic screening. Standardly, this involves a single x-ray of the breasts a medio-lateral view, although it is also possible for it to involve a double x-ray (both medio-lateral and cranio-caudal). Of course, the double x-ray procedure is more expensive, and most trials testing breast cancer screening by this method in fact relied simply on the medio-lateral views. These x-rays (or mammograms) are then sent to radiologists for interpretation. It is important to note here that the word 'interpretation' is appropriate. The mammograms do not detect cancer as such. What they detect is tissue abnormalities. But whether these abnormalities will develop into tumours its not revealed by the mammograms.

25

Nor do they reveal if any tumours detected are malign or benignant.

If an abnormality shows up on the first mammogram, the radiologist has to exercise her judgement as to the appropriate course of action. If she thinks for any reason that the abnormality is not worth pursing, the woman will hear no more. If on the other hand, the radiologist thinks that the abnormality is suspicious, then the woman will be invited back for a screening, knowing that breast cancer is suspected. If the second mammogram reveals the same abnormality, the next step is a biopsy to reveal the nature of the abnormality.

Screening by mammography thus appeared an attractive option, promising diagnoses early enough to obviate the need for major surgery. Furthermore, there had been a number of trials overseas which looked promising; and we now turn to consider the evidence which these trials provided in support of the practice of screening.

5 Evidence appearing to support mammographic screening

At the time that the Forrest Committee were deliberating, a number of clinical trials had been completed in Europe. The results of some of these trials had been apparently promising, and were used as evidence to support the recommendations that the Committee finally made. However, almost all of the studies, particularly those which claimed the best results, have been highly criticised, and have therefore been the source of great controversy concerning the validity of their results. It is therefore necessary to look in some detail at these studies, and at the criticisms of them.

a The HIP trial

The earliest controlled trial of breast cancer screening using mammography was the Health Insurance Plan trial, commonly referred to as the HIP trial (Shapiro, 1991), which was launched in December 1963, by Shapiro and colleagues at the Cancer National Institute in America. The purpose of the trial was to determine whether, by detecting breast cancer at an earlier, pre-clinical phase, using periodic breast cancer screening by mammography and clinical examination, mortality rates could be significantly effected.

Under the leadership of Michael Shimkin, who was at that time the director art the National Cancer Institute, it was decided that the trial should be conducted in New York, where a pre-paid medical care plan with about 700,000 members was in operation. This medical insurance plan had a computerised record system and had been previously engaged in epidemiological studies. One of the active members of this health plan was a radiologist: Phillip Strax who had been involved in the improvement of the mammographic technique.

Twenty three groups were chosen to take part in the study, each of these containing 80,300 women aged between 40 and 64 years of age. These groups were then stratified into five-year age cohorts, within which, every nth woman was allocated into the group which was to be screened, and every nth+1 woman was allocated into a control group and were not invited to be screened. Study and control group pairs were then randomly allocated into a sequence for the initial invitation to be screened. Active steps were taken to encourage women to attend for screening, and if the initial invitation was ignored then a follow up letter was sent, if this too was ignored then the woman was contacted by telephone. This very active approach produced a 67% response rate, and 20,000 women in the study group received an initial screen.

As it can be seen from the table (see Appendix 3), the screening procedure for this trial included clinical examination and a two-view mammography, (medio-lateral and cranio-caudal). All of the films were read and interpreted by two independent radiologists, with any differences of opinion being resolved by a third radiologist. Those women who had an abnormality reported, were referred to their group surgeon, and the subsequent identification of the biopsies and cancers diagnosed were made from the HIP records and hospital insurance claims. Deaths from breast cancer were ascertained by a follow-up of all cases diagnosed as breast cancer, contact with the patients family doctor and the death certificates. In order to counter possible inaccuracies in the death certificates, a verification procedure was used, and breast cancer deaths were defined as those deaths to which breast cancer was the underlying cause.

The authors of the report on the results of the trial were highly optimistic about the role of mammography in reducing the mortality from breast cancer. They reported an increased number of cancers in the study compared to the control group. But by five years after entry into the trial, the number of breast cancers in the study and control group was more or less equal, and at ten years after the trial had begun it was identical. After five years 304 cancers had been detected in the study group and 295 in the control group. As these patients had both clinical examination and a mammography, and these had been evaluated separately, it was possible to determine that had clinical examination not been included in the screening process, 45% of the cancers that had been detected would have been missed. However, compared to the control group, the women in the study group had tumours which were smaller and which had a reduced amount of lymph node involvement, and there was greater incidence of in situ disease.

After an analysis of the results from the trial, the authors reported a 30% reduction in mortality for the study group, and they claimed that this reduction in mortality emerged four years after the trial had begun. The conclusions of the report were:

The screening programme resulted in about a 30% reduction in mortality from breast cancer during the first ten years of follow up in the total group of study women aged 40-64 at entry. By the end of 18 years from entry, the reduction was about 25%. Accordingly, the HIP study provides strong evidence that periodic screening as conducted in this trial is indeed efficacious. Mammography was an important contributor to the reduction in breast cancer mortality. The issue that cannot be resolved, because of the joint application of mammography and clinical palpation, is the proportion of the decrease that can be attributed to this modality. (Wright, 1986, p. 1117)

b The Two Counties Trial

In addition to the evidence from the HIP trial, the Forrest Committee also used evidence from the so called 'Two Counties trial' in Sweden (Fagerberg, 1970). This trial was initiated by the National Board of Health and Welfare. It was to be a randomised trial of breast cancer screening using only single view mammography, and the trial was under the direction of Tabar and his colleagues. The trial included two counties in Sweden, Kopparberg and Oostergot land. Women living in the two counties were divided into 19 blocks according to their place of residence, and women were identified using the Swedish central population register, which is updated each year. In Kopparberg, each stratified group was divided into three groups for randomisation, two of the groups were allocated to be in the study group, while the other group were to be the control group. In Oostegotland, however, all of the groups were randomised into study and control groups.

All women in the study group were invited to come for screening by personal letter. The response to the letter varied across the age range of the women, with the group of women who were over 70 years of age responding so poorly that their results were eventually excluded from the report. Each woman in the control group who responded to the invitation to come forward for screening was given a single medio-lateral mammogram of each breast. For women who were aged between 40 and 49 years of age, the screening interval was two years, and for women who were aged 50 years or over, the screening interval was 33 months. All of the films were read by project radiologists, and where there were suspicious findings, the women were automatically recalled for a three view mammographic examination, if doubt remained, then she was referred for clinical examination, fine needle aspiration and cytology. Radiologists were responsible for the assessment procedure, and a surgeon was only involved if the radiologist thought that a biopsy was required.

In Sweden, a nation-wide cancer registration permits the easy identification of women who have developed breast cancer, including those who have moved out of the area. Deaths in both the study and the control groups were identified through the Central Bureau of Statistics.

The results of the trial published in 1984 showed a reduction in mortality of 31%. This was attributable, the authors thought, to both the high level of compliance, and the stage at which the cancer was detected. The authors claimed that there had been a marked shift towards the discovery of cancers at a more manageable stage, ie at an earlier stage. They claimed that in the study group, cancers were of a smaller size when discovered and had reduced axillary involvement compared to women in the control group.

c The TEDBC trials

A number of trials had been going on in the UK during the 70s and 80s. In the 1970s a few pilot centres had been set up, and three or four of these had been designated to determine the feasibility of screening for breast cancer using mammography. It was recognised that there was a need to evaluate the possibility of screening for breast cancer within the confines of the National Health Service, and it was with this in mind that a working group was created under the chairmanship of Sir Richard Doll, which planned a comparative study of the mortality rates of breast cancer in the various health districts which offered different services for the early detection of breast cancer. The study was called the Trial of the early Detection of Breast Cancer, or the TEDBC.

Following requests for submissions, four health districts were chosen, two as screening districts using mammography, and these were Edinburgh and Guildford, and two were to screen for breast cancer using breast self examination techniques. Four comparison districts were identified as control areas, and these were Oxford, Dundee, Southmead and Stoke-on-Trent. In the screening districts, registers were compiled for all women between the ages of 45-64 from the lists of general practitioners, and this included those women who would reach the minimum age during the seven years that the trial was destined to take. Invitation to the screening centres was by personal letter. All women who attended the screening centres in Edinburgh and Guildford were given a clinical examination every year, with a mammogram in years one, three, five and seven. In Edinburgh, the initial mammographic screen was by two views, medio-lateral oblique and caudio-cranial, and on subsequent screens, women were given a single oblique view mammogram. In Guildford, a single oblique view was used for all screens. Breast cancers diagnosed were identified from the registers of histopathological findings of all of the biopsies performed by the trial pathologists.

The response to the initial round of screening was rather low, about 60% in Edinburgh and about 70% in Guildford, and by the time the final screening round had been reached this had fallen even further to 53% in Edinburgh and 65% in Guildford. Analysis of the results revealed that there had been no significant reduction in the mortality rates between the study districts and the control districts; and when the figures were stratified for age at death and the duration of the trial, mortality from breast cancer in the two screening districts combined was only reduced by 14% (UK Trial of Early Detection Of Breast Cancer Group,1988)

Edinburgh (Roberts, 1990), was one of the centres that had been chosen to test the viability of breast cancer screening using mammography with the NHS, and on the initiative of Professor Eric Samuel, a custom-built screening unit was built in the grounds of the community health centre. After the screening centre had been in operation for some time, discussions were initiated into the possibility of Edinburgh conducting a local controlled trial within the city of Edinburgh, and the idea was supported by the Cancer research Campaign and by the Chief Scientists Office of the Scottish Home and Health Department. At that time there had already been an active programme in the city of educating women in the art of breast self examination, and so it was felt that the Edinburgh project could very accurately determine the contributions to the early detection of breast cancer using clinical examination and mammography in these 'well informed' women. The randomisation of the women in the city was done according to the GP practice that a woman belonged to. Therefore, all of the women in a particular practice who were in the right age range were either allocated into the study group or into the control group, and women were invited to the screening centre by personal letters. As with the TEDBC, all of the women in the control group received a clinical examination. At the first screen women received a two view mammogram, but at all subsequent screening rounds a single oblique view was given. The identification of breast cancer was identical to the TEDBC trial, and deaths were notified from the General Registry Office in Edinburgh. Perhaps not surprisingly, the results of the Edinburgh trial were identical to the results of the TEDBC, and were not statistically significant.

Early on in the study it was appreciated that the fact that women had been randomised according to their doctors practices may have had a confounding influence on the results of the trials, since the socio-economic status effected not only the attendance of women to the screening centres, but also affected the mortality rates, and a study carried out by Alexander and her colleagues between practices showed that mortality rates differed considerably between practices. The blame for the poor results of the UK trial has also been placed in the inaccuracies of the FPC records, and upon the poor compliance of British women.

We can thus see that not only was it the case that the major weaknesses of the early treatment of breast cancer had created a demand for improved diagnosis and treatment; it was also the case that a variety of trials appeared to show that breast cancer screening was exactly the procedure that was being sought. However, as we shall now go on to show, this comforting picture is entirely misleading.

6 Critique of the pro-screening evidence

In spite of the fact that the 'successful' trials seemed to provide convincing evidence in support of screening, there were serious problems with them, either in the design of the trial itself, or in the interpretation of the results. In this section, we shall focus on two of the most high-profile trials, and show why they do not really show what they seem to show.

a The HIP trial re-evaluated

In a critique of the HIP trial Haagensen and Asch (1986), have pointed out that the inclusion of mammography would account for the prevention of only three deaths in seven years. They also point out,

31

that according to their analysis only 0.004% of the women screened using mammography benefitted from the technique. They also report that the 30% reduction in mortality that is claimed by the authors of the report is misleading. It actually only represents the prevention of one or two deaths per 10,000 women per year. They point out that there is an important difference between absolute benefit and the relative benefit of screening.

This point is taken up by Wright, a clinician who pointed out that the benefit gained by women from the reduction in mortality which is directly attributable to screening is about 0.01%. Therefore the net benefit in the HIP trial is:

> in terms of overall ten year mortality in the group offered mammography, was only 0.06%; that is overall mortality in the control group minus 6.82% in the study group, it is imperative that this 'absolute benefit' be quoted along with the relative '30% benefit' to women being invited for screening" (Wright, 1986, p. 1117)

The point is that even if there is a statistically significant result from a trial such as the HIP trial, then this would make very little clinical difference to any individual woman.

Another critic of the HIP trial, Petr Skrabanek points out that:

> There are many unexplained features in the HIP study; for example, breast cancer death reduction was observed only in years 4 to 6. This contradicts the theory of screening which expects a cumulative increase in the benefit because of early treatment of slowly growing tumours detected preferentially by mammography. There is a slight excess of breast cancers in the screened group (about 10-15%) which disappeared by year 5. The theory of screening would expect an accumulation of all excess cases at the first screen (due to early detection) and this excess should be carried over throughout the duration of the study. (Skrabanek, 1988, p. 92).

b The Two Counties trial re-evaluated

Of all of the studies that have been carried out on breast cancer screening using mammography, the Two Counties Trial has been one of the most influential and the most highly criticised. In an article published in Diagnostic Imaging, Petr Skrabanek outlines the main areas of criticism:

> The Swedish study has raised more questions than it has solved.
> The design of the study is unclear; in a series of publications by
> the researchers, the age range of the study population varied. The
> randomisation was based, not on individuals but on areas of
> residence. The Lancet paper provided no information on interval
> cancers and no overall mortality. Although the authors noted a
> 30% to 40% excess of breast cancers in the study group, this
> suggests overdiagnosis and overtreatment (Skrabanek, 1988, p. 93).

Skrabanek goes on to point out that on the basis of the
assessments made at the time of the mammography, quadrandecto-
mies were often performed with no other evidence of malignancy.
When urged by critics to release data on the overall mortality rates for
the Two Counties Trial, the authors finally released the information in
a letter to Lakarttiningen in Swedish. From this source it appears that
the overall mortality rate in the study group was slightly higher than
that in the control groups. Skrabanek therefore concludes that not a
single life was saved in more than half a million woman years
(Skrabanek,1989). He also points out that a disproportionate number of
women with breast cancer in the study group died causes other than
breast cancer, and that as the cause of death was not ascertained by
any independent pathologists, it might be more reliable to compare all
deaths in breast cancer cases regardless of the ascription on the death
certificate. When this is done, it has a dramatic effect on the apparent
benefit to women in the study group. Benefit is reduced in all of the
study groups, and in the Oostergotland arm of the study any benefit
disappears altogether. He comments:

> The so called 30% reduction claimed by the Swedish workers was
> the same as the benefit reported in the HIP trial, despite the fact that
> the compliance rate in Sweden was almost twice as good and the
> mammographic equipment was much more sophisticated. In
> absolute terms this 30% reduction (uncorrected for misdiagnosis),
> was 40 deaths less in 78,000 women screened in eight years, that is,
> one death less per 10,000 woman years (Anderson, 1988, p. 947).

One of the consequences of the high rate of false positives in the
Two Counties Trial is the huge increase in surgical interventions,
which includes biopsies and mastectomies. While the Two Counties
Trial was in progress, the rate of breast surgery in the study group

rose by about 75% and remained at that level for the entire observation period of seven years.

7 Evidence against screening

a The BCDPP trial

Not all the trials on screening by mammography yielded even prima facie support for the idea that such screening would be beneficial to women. A number of important studies indicated the opposite.

In 1973, the apparent benefits shown in the HIP study inspired the American Cancer Society, in association with the National Cancer Institute to initiate a large demonstration project to determine the feasibility of introducing mammographic screening on a nation-wide basis. The trial was called the Breast Cancer Detection Demonstration Project (BCDDP). In the original programme, 270,000 women were recruited into the screening programme, and some 27 centres throughout the United States were screening women using clinical examination and mammography every year. After five years, the recorded reduction in mortality was a disappointing 20%. As a follow up report, in 1982, the BCDDP published a summary report, (U.K. Trial of Early Detection of Breast Cancer Group, 1981), which sought to obtain an overview of the benefits of screening for breast cancer using the results of mammographic screening studies from several different trials.

Their conclusions were that 3.58% of the total number of women screened (ie 64% of the women with positive screening results) had been subjected to a biopsy of the breast, and that 0.54% of the total, or 9.8% of those with positive screens, were shown to have cancer. Therefore the false positive rate was approximately 4.99% of the total number of women screened, or 90% of those with positive screening results. Or to put it another way, 3.4% of the screened women who had had a biopsy performed, received a diagnosis of benign breast disease. The absolute reduction in the breast cancer mortality rate was 0.144% in the HIP study and 0.04% in the Swedish study. This could be stated in a different way: in the HIP study, one woman in every 694 derived actual benefit from the screening procedure in terms of increased survival from breast cancer, and in the case of the Swedish trial this figure falls to one woman in every 2,041 screened. If these figures are then designated as the actual benefit rate, then the ratio of harm to benefit for breast cancer screening ranges from 21:1 to 62:1.

In addition, the small reduction in deaths from breast cancer is not only lost but totally reversed in the total mortality rates because of the increased deaths from other causes. The authors of the report remark that:

> Another disturbing feature of the results is the inclusion of cases of carcinoma in situ as 'cancers' found by screening. it is well known that only 50% of women with duct carcinoma in situ, and 20% of those with the lobular type will have invasive cancer. In other words, most women with carcinoma in situ of the breast, do not subsequently have breast cancer at all. This fact together with the lead time bias in any screening programme, renders the measure of case survival rates of no interest at all, and yet reports of the HIP study continue to publish impressive looking graphs of case survival rates (UK Trial of Early Detection of Cancer Group, 1988, p. 414)

Under a section headed "Harm/benefit Assessment", the authors of this report comment on the positive side of the balance sheet there is a marginal reduction in the deaths from breast cancer in older women, but on the negative side, is the financial cost and the induced morbidity. Negative factors also include the false positive results which lead to unnecessary surgery, the false negative rate which lead to inappropriate reassurance, and the raised level of anxiety in the female population, plus the risk of radiation induced cancers. The authors therefore conclude that:

> With the present evidence of benefit and current mammographic techniques, screening should only be offered to those women at high risk of developing breast cancer, for example those with a strong female history or with lobular carcinoma in situ (p. 115)

b The Canadian trial

A second important study whose findings went against the thesis that universal screening by mammography was beneficial was started in Canada in 1980. Its design was strongly influenced by the results just then emerging from the HIP trial in America, and also by the review of the United States Breast Cancer Demonstration Projects (BCDDP). The Canadian study commenced in January 1980. The screening examinations were initially planned to be conducted annually over a period of four years, but in order to set a termination date, the organisers of the study decided that women who had been recruited towards the end of the recruitment phase would be offered a total of four screens, as in the HIP study. The trial was conducted in Toronto and Vancouver. In order to ensure a good response to the invitation to be screened it was decided that a multiplicity of recruitment measures should be used to bring women to the screening centre, where they would be randomised after providing informed consent. This decision meant that all of the women had to be offered at least one mammogram. All of the women in the study group were given a mammography plus a clinical examination. They were also taught how to examine their own breasts. It was planned to recruit about 90,000 women into the project. The two view mammography (cranio-caudal and medio-lateral) was used initially, but after the recruitment had been completed, the medio-lateral projection was replaced by the medio-lateral oblique in all but two centres.

The results of the Canadian trial were very disappointing, and the authors were cautious about publishing the full findings:

> A decision has been taken by our Policy Advisory Group that cancer detection rates by modality should not be published as they might be misrepresented by the uninitiated (Miller, 1980, p. 107)

In their discussion of the results of the trial, there was considerable caution concerning the advantages of implementing breast cancer screening using mammography as a preventive measure:

> In conclusion, breast cancer screening requires continued evaluation and cannot currently be adopted as a population manoeuvre. Our present difficulties have partly arisen from the fact that assumptions are being made over the benefit from improving technology that have not so far been established. It has not been established that a significant mortality reduction follows from the earlier detection of such cancers, and only the NBSS has been designed to answer this question — and that only in women aged between 50-59. We are beyond the stage when large scale population screening programmes for cancer or indeed any disease should be introduced on the basis of assumed benefits. In our view the benefits of initiating mammographic screening in women and of adding mammography to the skilled examination of the breasts, have not yet been established. One final note of caution: if the major benefit in women aged 50 or more in the HIP study derived from the physical examination component of the screen, the benefit to be derived from the addition of mammography to the procedure would be minimal (Miller, 1980, p. 110)

Partly in response to some methodological criticisms (which we outline below) of the Two Counties Trial, another Swedish trial was launched, this time in Malmo, by Andersson and his colleagues. (Andersson, 1988). In this trial women who were aged between 40 and 70 years of age were identified through the population register and divided into 25 birth year cohorts. Within each of the birth year cohort groups women were randomly divided into study and control groups. Those who were to be screened received a personal letter. Women who refused the first invitation were invited to subsequent screens only if the lived in Malmo. In this study, each woman in the study group received a two view (medio-oblique and cranio-caudal) mammogram.

In Malmo there was one general hospital where a specialist team treated according to a standard policy protocol, almost all of the breast cancers in the city. Those women who required a biopsy were referred to this team who treated not just the women in the study group, but also those in the control group. The number of deaths and the causes of deaths were ascertained through the National Cancer Registry, and included those women who had moved out of the city. 76% of recorded breast cancer deaths in both the study and the control groups, had post mortem examinations to verify the cause of death.

The results of this trial were less encouraging than the results from the Two Counties Trial, and the reduction in the mortality rates were not statistically significant. An excess of cancers was again found in the first round of screening, and this excess persisted until the end of the trial eight years later. More non-invasive cancers were detected in the study than in the control group and the cumulative rate of stage II and more advanced cancers followed the same pattern as the Two Counties Trial. The overall result of the trial was that there was no significant reduction in breast cancer mortality in women in the study group. In fact it exceeded the number of deaths in the control group during the first six years of the trial.

However, the poor results were not regarded by the experimenters as good evidence against the efficacy of the screening programme. Rather, the results were explained by appealing to the fact that although the control populations in the study were not invited for periodic screening, there existed a policy of free access to breast screening. After the Malmo trial a survey of 500 women who had been involved in the trial revealed that 24% of them had gone for at least one mammogram at a centre other than the trial one.

d The Stockholm trial

Yet another trial in Sweden, this time in Stockholm (Frossell, 1989) in March of 1981, produced similar results, in this trial, as with the Malmo trial, women were individually randomised into control group and study group, and all of the women in the study group were given a single view (oblique) mammogram. By 1985, two full screening rounds had been completed. The results so far are inconclusive, as no overall mortality figures are yet available. But, as with the previous Swedish trial, the cumulative breast cancer rate at the five year stage in the study group, exceeded that of women in the control group by about 4%.

e The Nijmegen trial

Sweden was not the only place where controlled trials were taking place. In 1975, a trial was launched in the Netherlands (Verbeek, 1984). This was a population based breast cancer screening trial. Single view oblique mammography was used as the only screening examination every two years. In the first screening round, all women living in Nijmegen who were aged between 35 and 65 were invited to take part. In all four screening rounds were completed. The results showed that despite the breast screening there had been:

> No fall in the breast cancer mortality rate in Nijmegen up to the end of 1981 . . . Early treatment of breast cancer may not influence the chance of recovery, but may merely postpone the death due to breast cancer (p. 26)

The authors also recognised that there were problems associated with false negatives, two thirds of which were due to the fact that fast growing tumours were undetected at the times of screening, and this was demonstrated by the fact that a high percentage of the women who died of breast cancer during the course of the trial, died as a result of breast cancers which developed between the screening rounds.

8 Discussion in the medical journals

Though there were hints of controversy over the value of a breast cancer screening programme in the lay press, there were more obvious examples of the difference of opinion among members of the medical community. A good illustration of this is a series of letters in the *British Medical Journal* that appeared in the autumn of 1989. A heated exchange of views was provoked by an article written by Dr Maureen Roberts. Dr Maureen Roberts was the clinical director of the Edinburgh Breast Screening Project from 1979 until June of 1989, when she died of breast cancer. She was also one of the consulting experts used by the Forrest Committee. Her article, published six months after her death, revealed that she had many reservations and doubts concerning the effectiveness of a national breast cancer screening programme:

> We all know that mammography is an unsuitable screening test it is technologically difficult to perform, the pictures are difficult to interpret, it has a high false positive rate, and we don't know how often to carry it out. We can no longer ignore the possibility that screening may not reduce mortality in women of any age, however disappointing this may be (Roberts, 1989, p. 1336).

The reasons she gives for this conclusion are very detailed. She points out that the number of women who are likely to benefit each year from the breast cancer screening programme is very small. She gives the example from the Edinburgh project. For every 2,400 new patients with breast cancer seen each year in Scotland, 800 are aged 50-64, which is the age range specified by the Forrest Committee, who should be routinely screened. Of this 800, 270 will be invited for screening, 180 of these will attend the clinic or screening centre and 54 of these will benefit if there is a 30% reduction in mortality. But, together with her doubts about the benefits that women are likely, or unlikely to gain from the process of breast cancer screening using mammography, she also expressed a worry that the screening process might actually be detrimental. This is in part due to the false positive rate, but it is mostly due to the fact that there is no clear agreement between clinicians about how the disease should be managed — especially in the case of non-invasive carcinoma in situ. Given these problems, she felt that screening centres should at least be honest with the women who attend, both about the benefits and the possible problems with the procedure:

> They [women] should be told that the test is to detect cancer while it is still small; that we don't know how much it can influence mortality but there is up to a 30% chance (though it may be much less) that it may prolong life; that the test does not

39

detect all cancers, some of which may appear in the next three years; it can indicate only what the breasts are like today and cannot predict whether breast cancer will develop in the future. In addition, we do not know how to treat breast cancer. There is no successful treatment; different surgeons will carry out different procedures. Only a minority of women will be given this result however, and those who are normal can feel suitable reassured - except that they can develop the disease at any time: screening is not prevention (Roberts, 1989, p. 1336)

Finally she makes to point that the introduction of the screening programme was not based entirely on medical evidence, rather it was a decision made for purely political reasons. She comments on the willingness of the government to pour money into the breast cancer screening programme, while at the same time it is very unwilling to take on the tobacco industry at a political level, despite the overwhelming evidence that a truly preventive programme would save thousands of lives each year from lung cancer and other smoking related diseases. She comments:

It was clearly a matter of politics, a decision taken in an election year and now out of perspective. (Roberts, 1989, p. 1336)

Her article provoked a flurry of letters to the *British Medical Journal*, some supporting her views and others claiming that she was wrong in both of her conclusions and in her use of evidence from the trials. This correspondence gives an indication of the kinds of arguments used in the debate for and against the programme, and it might therefore be useful to look fairly closely at it.

One of the longest letters in reply to Dr Roberts came from Dr Jocelyn Chamberlain who was a member of the Forrest Committee, and was later a member of the advisory committee. Her rebuttal of Maureen Roberts's position was based on the proposition that screening for breast cancer using mammography had a sound statistical basis, and also that recent studies had supported the decision to implement the recommendations of the Forrest Committee. She agreed with Dr Roberts that there might be a slight risk of over diagnosis, but thought that this was simply the price we have to pay for a test which is sufficiently sensitive to pick up progressive cancer at a stage where it is still curable. (Chamberlain, 1989, p. 1192)

Others supported Dr Roberts, but on slightly different grounds. Dr Hewitt, for example suggested that from a biological standpoint it is almost impossible to detect a cancer at an early enough point in time:

> If we assume exponential growth of a tumour volume doubling time of two months, a tumour of only 2mm diameter will have been resident in the tissues for about three years and eight months and will contain about four million cells; by the time it reaches 3cm diameter it will have been resident for about five years seven months. Thus, a tumour diagnosed by screening at the smallest possible size detectable will already have gone through 65% of the time taken to reach a size that is easily palpable. Clearly screening is far from capable of *early* diagnosis. (Hewitt, 1989, p. 1337)

The point that Dr Hewitt is making is that if death from breast cancer is most often associated with disseminated disease, then the apparent earlier diagnosis possible through screening with mammography would not be expected to effect long term mortality.

Another writer, Dr Ashworth broadly agrees with Dr Hewitt concerning the problems of how 'early' is early enough in biological terms, and then goes on to conclude, as did Dr Roberts that based on the evidence:

> The decision to embark on breast cancer screening has been based on political and not medical grounds" (Ashworth, 1989, p. 1337).

Others were not quite so negative about the programme — mainly on the grounds that although there were problems with it, having got a national programme, we might as well make the most of it. Dr Ruth Ellman who, like Jocelyn Chamberlain, was a member of the Forrest Committee, commented that:

> I share Maureen Roberts's opinion that the introduction of the breast cancer screening programme was overhasty, but the situation will not be improved by abandoning public screening. (Ellman, 1989, p. 1337)

Other writers echoed this thought, Dr Ashbury, for example wrote:

> Many of us do fear that the screening programme will ultimately

fail in Britain, not least because of the inadequacies of Family Practitioner Committee registers and the lack of 'compliance' of British women; but let us at least give it a good try (Ashbury, 1989, p. 1337)

This brief look at the letters column of the *British Medical Journal* in November of 1989 represents a sort of snapshot of the kinds of debates taking place around the issue of breast cancer screening. But the controversy was much more wide ranging than this might suggest. There were a whole series of objections to the programme which were both from within and outside the programme, and on a whole variety of grounds.

9 Other problems with screening

a The radiation danger

One of the disadvantages with the early techniques of mammography, was that although reasonably good views might be obtained, the dose of radiation to the breast required to breast required to produces the image was excessive. By 1976, there was considerable concern that the mammogram might be an actual initiator of cancer of the breast. The evidence for this came not from women who had been subjected to radiation through mammography, but on evidence from a study carried out on women (or girls) who received doses of radiation after an atomic explosion (Tokunga, 1984; Modan et al., 1989; Boice 1979; Kamadia, 1968; Cohegan, 1986; Modan et al., 1979). The females involved had been aged between 14 and 15 years of age at the time of the atomic explosion at Hiroshima. The study only included 28 survivors, and of these, six had developed breast cancer. This report, as well as several others, suggested that breast tissue was particularly susceptible to the effects of radiation, and that this was especially pronounced in women who were under 20 years of age. Another more recent report from Israel also indicates that low-dose irradiation of even younger females (aged 5-9 years) significantly effects their risk of developing breast cancer later in life.

At high levels of radiation, the relationship between dose and effect is far more clear, and obviously linear. it was therefore essential that it be discovered whether the relatively low doses associated with mammography posed a serious risk to the patient. In order to determine this, one method was to extrapolate the dose effect curve, and another was to consider the results of experimental work, which had been done using animals. On the basis of the evidence, it appeared to some at least, that the radiation risk associated with mammography was very low:

> This evidence suggests that if two million women over the age of 50 were to receive a low-dose single view mammogram, there would be, after a latent period of ten years, one excess cancer per year. Compared to an incidence of breast cancer at age 60 that approaches 2000 per million women, this risk is of no consequence. (Forrest, 1986, p. 81)

But despite the willingness of the Forrest Committee to dismiss the suggestion that screening with mammography might constitute an acceptable risk, others have suggested that the risk to women from the radiation is only 'of no consequence' if the woman is presenting with *symptomatic* breast disease. The risk to women who are *symptomless* is quite another matter, especially if the intention is to set up a national screening programme where millions of such women will be subjected to a mammogram every year.

b Sensitivity versus specificity

Screening healthy women using mammography has one clear aim, and that is to detect occult breast cancer. In order to do this, the radiologist has to determine whether the films are normal or test negative, abnormal or test positive, or are of a quality that does not allow clear interpretation. In order that screening mammography can achieve its aims, it is important that the test is both *sensitive* and *specific*. It is also important that it has a good *predictive value*.

The sensitivity of screening mammography defines the proportion of women who have cancer of the breast and for whom a positive test result is recorded. That is, that the cancer has been correctly detected by the mammogram. To calculate sensitivity, it is necessary to know the number of women who are test positive and those who are falsely diagnosed as test negative, so that the total number of breast cancer cases can be calculated. But this can only be accurately determined if every woman who has received a test negative result is fully investigated, which would ideally need to include a biopsy of both breasts. This would clearly not be an acceptable course of action. For this reason, the number of interval cancers which emerge after a year is taken to be the number of cancers missed by the initial screening round.

Specificity, is the extent to which a positive or abnormal mammogram is recorded in women who do not have breast cancer. In other words, a false positive result. Petr Skrabanek has challenged the validity of the breast cancer screening programme on the grounds that it fails to satisfy any of the above criteria:

> Mammography is not a good screening test, since its positive predictive value in symptomatic populations is low. In the Canadian Breast Cancer Screening Study (still in progress), the positive predictive value was 8.6% (range 3-16% in five different screening centres); that means that out of every 100 positive mammograms, 84 to 97 are false positives (Baines et al., 1986). Mammography also has low sensitivity. Even cancers large enough to be palpable are often missed by mammography. For example, in a recent series of 139 palpable tumours in women under the age of 51, 44% were false negatives. The range of sensitivity in various mammographic screening programmes was 29% to 69%, with a mean of 60%. While sensitivity has improved with more advanced technology, the low specificity of mammography is a cause for serious concern. Using a specificity of 92% as obtained recently at the Royal Marsden Hospital, and assuming a prevalence of breast cancer of 3 per 1000 after the first screen, the implementation of the Forrest Report would result in over 100,000 false positive mammograms a year (Skrabanek, 1988, p. 116).

However, as Forrest himself has pointed out (Forrest, 1990), it is very difficult for any screening test to be both highly sensitive and highly specific as to some extent they are inversely related to each other. This is because where the radiologist 'draws the line' turns out to be of vital importance. If the line of suspicion is set very high in order that every abnormal film is investigated further, this means that a large number of women who do not have breast cancer will be recalled needlessly, in which case the specificity will be very low. On the other hand, if the radiologist adopts a more relaxed attitude to apparent abnormalities, then more cases of cancer are missed. So while the test may be more specific, the sensitivity of the test will be much lower. Skrabanek says that this dilemma is based upon the fact that mammography is simply not very good at distinguishing between cancer and non-cancer, and it is therefore necessary to confirm findings with a biopsy. The smaller the abnormality, then the more

44

difficult the job of the radiologist becomes:

> Once women start asking questions with medic-legal implica-
> tions, radiologists will be under pressure to cover themselves by
> overinterpreting mammographical findings. This will be a parti-
> cular problem in the grey area of impalpable lesions grouped
> under such vague terms as occult cancer, minimal breast cancer,
> pre-cancer, carcinoma in situ, atypical hyperplasia, borderline
> lesions etc, which present a potential for mis-diagnosis. Even in
> relatively straight forward intra-ductal carcinoma in situ, the
> natural history is poorly understood and only a minority of such
> lesions would progress to invasion if left alone; in the case of
> lobular carcinoma in situ, the treatment option range from doing
> nothing to bilateral prophylactic mastectomy (Skrabanek, 1989, p.
> 479).

Other writers have also noticed this tendency, and have
commented upon its possible consequences. At the Los Angeles
Conference on breast cancer, Gold remarked:

> Lesions that are not malignant and never will be are sometimes
> diagnosed as early cancer . . . such overdiagnosis not only
> increases the number of cancers detected, but can inflate the
> number of cancers detected in the earliest stages. Because these
> lesions never become clinically significant, survival statistics may
> also appear improved. (Gold, 1988, p. 47).

Another problem associated with the sensitivity and specificity of
the mammogram is that the films require a high degree of skill to read.
Unlike an x-ray of a broken bone, a small lesion is not obvious. The
picture requires experienced and skilled interpretation. Isobel Furnival
et al. (1970) reported that in a study of the ways in which radiologists
interpret mammograms revealed that there was a considerable amount
of disagreement between radiologists over the interpretations of
mammograms. Their study involved three radiologists examining the
mammograms of 477 patients, they found that:

> There was considerable disagreement between the three radiolo-
> gists . . . though at least one noted malignant disease in 56
> women, in only nine cases was there agreement between two of
> the observers, and in only two cases was there agreement
> between all three. In none of the 70-mm mammograms reported

as malignant did two or all three of the radiologists agree on a diagnosis. (p. 47)

They therefore concluded that:

All three radiologists agreed in less than one third of the cases. A single radiologist reporting on either a thermogram or a mammogram film is likely to be inaccurate in a significant proportion of cases . . . The incidence of false positive reports as assessed in patients with benign disease and in asymptomatic women is high. (Furnival, 1970, p. 49)

The authors of this report felt that the sensitivity and specificity of mammograms was so low, and that the amount of reader error was so high, that mammography should not be used as a screening tool, especially if it was to be the only screening tool. In fact they commented that it would be 'dangerous' to use mammography as a single screening modality as it would lead either to overdiagnosis or to a false sense of security in the patient.

c Is early diagnosis always desirable?

Last but not least, is the controversy surrounding the notion that an earlier diagnosis of breast cancer always leads to an improved diagnosis, and indeed, if the cancer is caught at an early enough stage, then a cure is possible, or even probable. It is essential for screening to be effective that this earlier diagnosis should lead to an improved prognosis, otherwise there is no point to it at all.

There is, however, some evidence to suggest that this might not be the case. It is not the timing of the discovery that is the most important factor in the prognosis, by the biological type of the neoplasm. Skrabanek points out that with reference to BSE (breast self examination), this is the reason poor results have been gained from teaching women to examine their own breasts:

Failure to accept this reality is the main reason that the futile and bitter dispute between radicalists and conservationists remains unresolved. The radicalist wing proposes more extensive surgery for carcinoma in situ or stage I tumours than for tumours with axillary or systemic metastases. This puts the woman who has been practising BSE, or who has been invited to attend mass mammography screening into the unenviable position: earlier detection may lead to more extensive surgery (Skrabanek, 1988, p. 97)

The evidence that a shift in the time of the diagnosis always leads to an improved prognosis, therefore is far from conclusive in the case of breast cancer. Skrabanek, (and others) have pointed to the biological natural history of a tumour. Even a tumour that is very small, has already been growing for eight to twelve years and has had ample opportunity to metastasize, or disseminate. Indeed it has been found that in all of the controlled trials, a large proportion of the cancers found have had nodal involvement.

From all of the above, it can be seen that there is a considerable amount of controversy over almost every single aspect of the screening of symptomless women for breast cancer. But the response of the advocates of the screening programme is clear. Moskowitz (1987) says that the questions that are constantly being raised by those who question the wisdom of the screening programme are best answered if the critics undertook some studies themselves:

> The scientific shoe is now on the other foot. Its no longer up to me or anyone else who support screening to prove its effectiveness. Those who don't believe must set up a similar trial, and if after fifteen years they fail to show any tendency to benefit, then I would have to say I might be wrong. (1979, p. 72)

But there seem to be little chance of the critics engaging in such a trial. Given, therefore, the above controversy within the medical world, one is drawn more and more towards the conclusion stated by Dr Roberts that the decision to implement a national breast cancer screening programme is not a decision which rests purely and simply upon clear medical evidence of its benefits. It is much more likely to have been a decision based on political expediency.

10 Summary of objections

Drawing together the objections to the screening programme which have been expressed, we can summarise them as follows:

1 Mammography is not an effective screening test. It cannot find a satisfactory midpoint between high levels of false negatives and false positives. The false negatives mean that there are many

women who have cancer who will not be identified by the screening. The false positives mean that many women who are not in fact ill will have been called back for further screening, for biopsies, and even breast surgery assessment, with all the high levels of anxiety that this can cause, both for the women themselves and for their families.

2 A negative screening has no predictive value: it does not imply that the patient will not develop cancer in the future, even on the day after the screening. So to be effective the screening needs to occur regularly. But there is some evidence that repeated exposure to low dose radiation can actually *cause* breast cancer (Modan et al., 1989)

3 The claim that screening programmes can improve mortality rates is at best poorly supported by the evidence from some trials, while other trials actually suggest the opposite.

4 The decision to implement the Forrest recommendations was premature. The results of the UK trial were still awaited, and there was no point in setting up the trial in the first place, if its findings were to be pre-dated by the Committee's recommendations.

5 Breast cancer screening using mammography is expensive, time consuming and difficult. The money would be more productively used if it were spent on researching into the underlying causes of cancer.

What has become clear from the preceding discussion is there did not exist the medical consensus that many individuals and groups thought there was concerning the usefulness of breast cancer screening using mammography. Moreover, it has been argued by some that the net result of screening with mammography is that it does more harm than good. This leads us to ponder first, on why the Forrest Committee so enthusiastically supported a national programme — since, unlike the lay public they would (at the very least) been aware of the controversy which surrounded it; and secondly on why the government were willing to commit large amounts of public money to a programme which was based on equivocal medical evidence.

In the following chapter we shall be considering how a 'rationalist' approach to decision making might provide us with an analytical framework through which the actions of the Forrest Committee might be understood. In order to do this, we will be examining the various varieties of rational actor models and attempt to apply each of them to the case study of breast cancer screening.

References

Anderson, I., Aspagen, K., Janson, L., et al., (1988); 'Mammographic Screening and mortality from Breast Cancer: The Malmo Mammographic Screening Trial', *The British Medical Journal*, vol 297, pp. 943-948.

Ashbury, D., (1989); Correspondence, *The British Medical Journal*, vol 299, p. 1337.

Ashworth, T., (1989); Correspondence, *The British Medical Journal*, vol 299, p. 1337.

Baker, I., (1982); 'The Breast Cancer Demonstration Project: Five Year Preliminary Report', *Cancer*, vol 32, pp. 194-224.

Beatson, G., (1986); 'On The Treatment of Inoperable Cases of the Mamma' *The Lancet*, vol 12, pp. 104-7

Boice, T., Land, C., Shore, R., (1979); 'The Risk of Breast Cancer Following Low Dose Irradiation', *Radiology*, vol 131, pp. 589-97.

Brown, J., (1989); 'Rab and His Friends', Collected Papers, Cited in *Breast Cancer Screening*, Forrest, A., Nuffiield Trust, London.

Bunker, A.,. Baum, M, (eds); (1989); Mass Mammography — The Time for Reappraisal — Technology and Surgical Policy', *International Journal of Technology Assessment in Health Care*, Special Issue, Spring.

Cohegan, J., Darby, W., Spitznagal, et al., (1988); 'Radiogenic Breast Cancer, Effects of Mammographic Screening' *The Journal of the National Cancer Institute*, vol 77, pp. 71-76.

Davey, J., Greening, W and McKinna, J; (1970), 'Is Screening for Cancer Worthwhile?', *British Medical Journal*, 19th Sept, pp. 696-699.

Day, M, and Miller, A, B., (1986); 'Canadian National Breast Screening Study' in *Screening For Breast Cancer*, Hans Huber Publishers, Toronto.

Dixon, T., (1974); 'Breast Cancer, The Debate Continues', *The Canadian Family Physician*, vol 116, pp. 187-190.

Dowle, C, S., and Blamey, R., et al., (1970); 'Preliminary Results of the Nottingham Breast Self Examination Education Programme', British Journal of Surgery vol 74, pp. 217-219.

Early Breast Cancer Trials Group, (1985); 'The Effects of Adjuvant Tamoxifen and of Cytotoxic Therapy on Mortality in Early Breast Cancer. An Overview of 61 Randomised Controlled Trials among 28,896 women', The New England Journal of Medicine, part 4, pp.125-133.

Ellman, Ruth., (1987); Correspondence, *The British Medical Journal*, vol 299, p. 1337.

Ellman, Ruth., (1987); 'A Cautious Two Cheers For Screening' *Preventive Medicine*, February, p. 3.

Fentman, I., (1988): 'Pensive Women and Painful Vigils', *The Lancet*, vol 1, pp. 1041-2.

Forrest, A, P., (1989); 'A Lister Oration: Breast Cancer 121 Years on'. *The Journal of the Royal College of Surgeons*, vol 34, pp. 239-48.

Forrest, A, P., (1986); *Breast Cancer Screening: Report to the Health Ministers of England and Wales*, HMSO, London.

Forrest, A, P., (1990); *Breast Cancer: The Decision To Screen*, Nuffield Provincial Hospitals Trust, London.

Frank,. (1985); 'Breast Self-examination, More Harm Than Good?', *The Lancet*, vol 2, pp. 654-657.

Frissel, J., Hellstrom, L., et al.; (1989); 'The Stockholm Breast Cancer Screening Trial — Five Year Results and State at Discovery'. *Breast Cancer Research and Treatment*, vol 13, pp. 79-87.

Frissel, J., Hellstrom, L., et al., (1987); 'A Randomised Trial For Breast Cancer in Stockholm', *Breast Cancer Research and Treatment*, vol 8, pp. 45-45

Furnival, I., Stewart, H., Weddall, J., (1970); 'Accuracy of Screening Methods For the Diagnosis of Breast Disease', *British Medical Journal*, 21st Nov, pp. 47-8.

Gold., (1988)., (1988); 'Analysis: The Screeners', *Diagnostic Imaging*, vol 4, no 3, p. 47.

Halstead, W, S., (1907); 'The Results of Radical Operations For The Cure of Carcinoma of the Breast', *Journal of Surgery*, vol 49, pp. 1-19.

Hewitt, H., (1989); Correspondence, *British Medical Journal*, vol 299, p. 1337.

Hill, D., (1987); 'Self-Examination, Is It Beneficial?' *British Medical Journal*, vol1 297, 23rd July.

Hobbs, P., (1985); 'The Use of Breast Self-examination as a Screening Modality' *Journal of the Institute of Health Education*, vol 23, part 4, pp. 125-133.

Kamadia, N., Stigera, C., Kuratoto, A., et al. (1968); 'Acute and Late Effects of a Bomb Radiation; Studied in a Group of Young Girls with a Defined Condition at the Time of Bombing', *The Journal of the National Cancer Institute*, vol 77, pp. 71-76.

MacGuire, T., Lee, E., (1978); 'Psychiatric Problems in The Year After Mastectomy', *British Medical Journal* vol1, pp. 963-5.

Makowitz., (1979); 'Cost Benefits Determinants in Screening Mammography', *Cancer*, October 1st.

Miller, A., (1980); 'The Canadian National Breast Screening Study',

Screening For Breast Cancer, Day and Miller (eds), Huber Publishers, Toronto, Canada.

Modan, B., Cherit, A., Alfandry, B and Katz,I., (1989); 'Increased Risk of Breast Cancer after Low Dose Irradiation', *The Lancet*, vol 1, 25th March, pp. 629-74.

Morris, T., Steven-Greer, H, J., (1977); 'Psychological and Social Adjustment to Mastectomy: A Two Year Follow up Study', *Cancer*, vol 40, pp. 2381-7

Radway, A., (1988); 'Breast Cancer Screening: A Continuous Controversy', *Cancer Topics*, vol 17, no 2, Sept/Oct.

Roberts, M., Alexander, F., Anderson, T., et al. (1990); 'The Edinburgh Trial of Screening for Breast Cancer', *The Lancet*, vol 1, pp. 1042-5.

Roberts, M., (1989); 'Breast Cancer Screening: Time For A Rethink?' *British Medical Journal*, vol 299, p. 1336.

Shapiro, S., Venet, W., Strax, P., Venet, L., (1991), 'Current Results of the Breast Cancer Screening Randomised Trials: The Health Insurance Plan of Greater New York Study', *Screening in Health Care*, Walter Holland and Susie Stuart (eds), The Nuffield Hospitals Provincial Trust, London.

Skrabanek, P., (1988), 'The Physicians Responsibility to the Patient', *The Lancet*, vol 1, 21st May, pp. 115-6.

Skrabanek, P., (1988); 'The Benefits of Mass Screening Rests on Equivocal Evidence', *Diagnostic Imaging International*, vol 4,no 3, June.

Skrabanek, P., (1989); 'Shadows Over Screening Mammography', *Clinical Radiology*, paper 479, vol 40.

Skrabanek, P., (1988); 'The Case Against', *The British Medical Journal*, 15th Oct, p. 971.

Skrabanek, P., (1989); 'Mass Mammography: A Time For Reappraisal', for Technology Assessment and Surgical Policy in *The International Journal of Technology Assessment in Health Care*, Special Spring Issue.

Skrabanek, P., (in Press); 'Breast Cancer Screening, A UK Showdown', *The British Journal of Hospital Medicine*.

Tabar, L., Fagerberg, C., Day, W., (1977); 'The Results of Periodic one-view Mammographic Screening in a Randomised Controlled Trial in Sweden' *Screening For Breast Cancer*, Day and Miller (eds) Huber Publishers, Toronto Canada.

Tokunga, M., L and, C., Yamamoto et al., (1984) 'Breast Cancer Among Atomic Bomb Survivors' *Radiation Carcinogenesis*, Boice and Faumani (eds), Raven Press, New York, pp. 124-30.

UK Trial of Early Detection of Breast Cancer Group, (1981); 'Trial of Early Detection of Breast Cancer: A Description of Method', *The British Journal of Cancer*, vol 44, pp. 618-27.

UK Trial of Early Detection of Breast Cancer Group, (1988); 'First Results on Mortality Reduction in the UK Trial Of Early Detection of Beast Cancer' The Lancet, vol 11, pp. 411-5.

Verbeek, A., Hendricks, J., et al., (1984); 'Reduction in Breast Cancer Mortality Through Mass Screening With Modern Mammography: The First Results of The Nijimegen Project', *Journal of Oncology*, vol 28, pp. 23-7.

Virchow, R., (1973); *Cellular Pathology*, Lipincott, London.

Vog Rosen, Frissell, Glans and Hellstrom et al., (1989); 'Non-palpable Invasive Breast Cancer From the Stockholm Screening Project', *Journal of Oncology*, vol 28, pp. 23-7.

Wright, C. J., (1986); 'Breast Cancer Screening, A Different Look at the Evidence', *Surgery*, vol 100, no 4.,

3 Rationalist theories of explanation

1 The benefits and dangers of explanatory models

What we have seen so far, is that the decision to implement a screening programme was not based simply on clear cut medical evidence. Given that this is the case, the task of this chapter is to examine ways in which political science has constructed models of decision making, in order to assist understanding of the processes involved. If such models are to be of any use, they must have explanatory scope; that is, that they must have broad application and they must also explain specific cases of decision making. In other words, if a model only helps us to understand one specific decision making process, or alternatively, is so vague that it does not offer any real insight, then the model might be considered to be deficient. In this chapter we will be examining various 'rationalist' approaches to the decision making process in order to discover if they may be of some use in the specific case of breast cancer screening.

Looking for the causes and the sources of public policies is an

53

occupation on which political scientists have expended a good deal of time and energy. Sometimes it has seemed that the issue under investigation is a fairly straightforward one, while at other times the researcher knows that the issue is far from simple. But in either case it usually transpires with elegant inevitability that the process of policy-making is highly complex, and at least on the surface, can appear noisy and chaotic. In order to try to bring some order to the appearance of muddle, many political scientists have tried to explain the processes of policy-making by developing and applying models which operationalise and structure the actions of the various actors concerned.

Although this approach has been useful and popular among political scientists, it also has its limitations. Once a model has been constructed and used as an explanatory framework, it tends to focus the attention of the researcher on certain areas while ignoring others. Rather like the drunk who looks for a lost key by the lamppost because the light is better there, so the researcher will be tempted to explain policy- making by reference to certain aspects of the process, or by reference to the actions of certain individuals or groups, because these are the aspects which are highlighted by that particular model. This then raises the problem that by illuminating certain aspects, other (and perhaps more important) aspects may be missed completely.

2 A pure rational actor model

Let us start with the rational actor (RA) model of traditional games theory. Immediately we need to notice two different ways in which such a theory can be interpreted. First, it may be interpreted in a normative way, as telling us not why we make the choices that we do, but only what we *ought* to do if we are to be rational. Alternatively, it could be read as an empirical theory, telling us why people do, in fact, do what they do. The difference between these is that on the first interpretation, if there is a mismatch between people's choices and the prescriptions of the theory, then it is the choices which are are at fault: the agents have not made the choices which they ought to have made. On the second interpretation, if there is a mismatch between the actual choices and the theory, then it is the theory which is at fault: it has failed to explain/predict the actual choices, and is thus in the same position as another empirical theory which generates failed explanations and/or predictions.

For our purposes, we shall adopt the second interpretation of the

RA theory. It will not matter from our point of view whether this is how most of its proponents intend it. We are simply asking the question 'Given that we wish to explain a piece of institutional decision-making by the Forrest Committee, could we explain it using the resources of RA accounts?' That this is not an arbitrary treatment of the theory is suggested by the fact that the members of the Forrest Commmitte themselves would doubtless have seen their decisions as a rational response to the problem with which they were confronted.

So what does an RA model look like? Let us start with the account provided by Hollis (1983) in *The Cunning of Reason*. Although Hollis is ultimately a critic of the theory, he nevertheless provides a sympathetic, lucid, and non-technical exposition of the theory's basic tenets. Consider, Adam in the Garden of Eden. Adam wants some mulberries and also wants some figs, but he wants the figs more, all other things being equal. So he gets himself some figs: he has been the archetypal rational actor who has maximised his preference satisfaction, or his utility. To this ultra simple model, complications can then be added. It may be that there are differential costs attached to meeting differetn satisfactions. Although Adam prefers figs to mulberries, the figs are very much further away, and require unpleasant exertions to obtain — exertions which are so unpleasant that he maximises his utility by settling for mulberries instead. It may be that he lacks total information about the consequences of his choices: although the mulberries wil be nearer if there are any, he is not absolutely certain that any still remain. If they *are* there, a journey to obtain will be a worthwhile cost; but if they already been eaten, the journey will be a cost which is not outweighed by any subsequent utility. So what he must aim to do is maximise his *expected* utility, while recognising that this may diverge considerably from his actual utility. Further complications appear in Adams' (rational) life with the arrival of Eve. In some situations, when he is calculating which action will maximise his expected utiltiy, he will have to take account of her likely behaviour. And in some situations, what she is likely to do may depend on what [she thinks] he is likely to do. Very much more refinement can be built into the model than this simply sketch includes. But this outline identifies for us the essential elements of the explanatory model. The rational actor must have an ordered set of preferences, she must have beliefs or information about the likelihood that any given action will lead to the satisfaction of her preferences, and her action can be explained by saying that she had just that set of preferences and that body of information, and she acted as she did *because* she had those preferences and that information.

3 Applying the RA model to the Forrest Committee

How, then, would this model apply to the Forrest Committee's decisions. Let us assume first of all that we can legitimately treat the Committee here as a single 'rational actor', and hence as having a single set of goals, and a shared body of information. This is a move which is fully within the traditions of the RA model — e.g. when for the purposes of the theory, firms are treated as 'rational actors' who are seeking to maximise their utility. But we should be clear that this *is* an assumption, and it is one which can be challenged. It overlooks the fact, for example, that if the Committee contained members with rival views, the shared pool of information might have been less than the information held by individual members. And it simply slides over the fact that the goals of the Committee may have been an unhappy compromise, the result of some conflict of goals among the members.

Given, however, that we are granting the legitimacy of applying the RA model to the deliberations of the Forrest Committee, there are are two ways in which the adequacy of the model can be tested. First, we could make assumptions about what the Committee's ordered set of preferences was; about the information which they had about the likelihood that various courses of action would maximise expected utility; and on the basis, predict what course of action the Committee would follow. If there is a mismatch between the predicted course of action and what the Committee actually did, that will be a disconfirmation of any claims by the RA theory to provide an adequate explantion.

Alternatively, we could start with the actual recommendations made by the Committee, and work back from them to what the ordered set of preferences, and the means-end information used by the Committee would have to be *if the RA theory is to be acceptable.* If it turns out that we cannot find any plausible candidates for either the preferences or the informatin, or both, then again the mismatch between theory and fact will be a disconfirmaton of the theory. (we emphasise again here the point which was made above: the RA theory is here being interpreted not as a normative theory prescribing what people ought to do if they are to be rational, but as an explanatory theory, purporting to explain why people do do what they do.)

Let us consider initially the first of the two routes described above. To begin with, we have to attribute to the Committee an ordered set of consistent preferences. To do this of course already to step into the field of interpretation. We can assume that their terms of reference provided them with some input into these preferences. But if

56

we are to apply the RA model, we need to assume a good deal more than just the terms of reference. Primarily, we need to assume that their dominant preference was the provision of the best practicable medical facilities for women in respect of breast cancer. In practice, of course this preference is qualified by other constraints on their decision-making. They must recognise that the resources that could be devoted to implementing any proposals they make are finite, and hence, other things being equal, they will prefer a cheaper treatment to a more expensive one. They know that they do not have endless time for their deliberations, and hence that they must attach some importance to the goal of completing the Report within a certain time span. Their dominant goal will obviously generate a number of other subgoals. For example, it would be reasonable to attribute to them the subgoal of wishing to acquire all the relevant scientific findings about the efficacy of the screening process, inthe light of which they could assess the likelihood of maximising the chances of realising their dominant goal. (The rational actor is rational in seeking to acquire relevant information, as well as in acting on it). And so on.

Let us take for granted, then, these background assumptions and assume that the dominant preference is the provision of the best practicable resources for breast cancer. Achieving that, we will assume, will yield maximum utility to the Committee.

What then of the information which determines the Committee's choice of means to achieve this maximum utility? Here we can be a little more specific than in relation to their preferences, because the Appendix to the Report lists the experimental studies, expert reports, etc. which the Committee relied on.

So what, on the basis of these preferences and this information, would the rational actor theory predict that the Committee would recommend? *If* the evidence had been solidly in favour of the benefits of the breast screening programme, we would have expected the Committee to make the recommendations which in fact they did make. But we have seen in Chapter 2 that the evidence was extremely equivocal. There *was* a consensus that the screening programme would be beneficial — but as we have seen, that was a consensus which existed much more in the popular mind than in the medical community. It is true that some studies (such as the HIP and Two Counties trials) had suggested that the screening programme would be very beneficial, with survival rates improving by up to 30%. But we have also seen how those studies were in fact deeply flawed.

Furthermore, again as Chapter 2 showed, there had been a number of trials which suggested that the screening had produced no improvement in mortality rates, and even in some cases that the mortality rate in the study group was *higher* than that in the control group!

In addition to this failure of trials to support the idea that a screening programme would improve mortality rates, there is the problem posed by 'false negatives'. Since these are women who turn out not to have cancer, they do not appear in any incidence or mortality statistics for the disease. But the alarm and despondency aroused in someone who is told that she may have breast cancer is nonetheless a major fact to be taken into account in determining the benefit to women of a test which yields a high number of false positives.

In the light of the problems posed by the screening programme which we described at length in the previous chapter, it is impossible to regard the Committee's recommendations as rational. Recommending nationwide-screening of symptomless women cannot be seen as providing the best practicable provision of facilities for coping with the disease.

What action or actions by the Committee *would* have been explained by the RA model? A full answer to that questin would take us beyond our present concerns. But it is worth considering the question briefly, in order to point out the divergence between the Committee's actual course of action and what a rational course of action would have been. We can thereby underline the inadequacies of the RA model. One obvious 'rational' course of action would have been to await the results from the lengthy UK trials which had started in 1979 and were due to be concluded in 1988. After all, Forrest himself and fourteen other members of the Forrest Committee had been involved in setting up and running the UK trial. Why should they think that suddenly its findings were no longer relevant - and come to that conclusion just as the trial was drawing to its close? It is not even as if the balance of evidence had swung heavily in favour of the screening programme after the UK trial was set up and before the Committee reported. As we saw when looking at the results of trials from elsewhere, the results were highly ambivalent. Surely, then, it would have eminently rational to recommend awaiting the results of the trial which they themselves had inaugurated.

Secondly, given some of the clearly identified problems with the screening programme (e.g. the problem of false positives), the Committee could have recommended that resources should be devoted to research designed specifically to rememdy this weakness in the programme. As was noted in Chapter 2, it had turned out to be impossible within the available technology to devise a test which was both specific and sensitive. Recommending further research in this area would have been a second course of action which, on the RA model, we might have expected the Committee to recommend.

There are then, at least two courses of action, quite different from those taken by the Committee, which would have had a better claim to be regarded as rational, and hence would have been predicted by the RA model. So if we take the second of the two routes which was outlined at the start of this section, we are forced to the conclusion that the Committee's actions cannot be explained on an RA account.

What, then, if we take the second of the two routes mentioned above — that is to say, we start with the Committee's recmmendations and work back from them to the information and preferences which, if the RA account were true, would have been what moved the Committee?

What are the striking features of the Committee's recommendations? What has so far been argued is one of the most striking features of the Committee's recommendations is that they were *not* in women's best interests. How, then, on an RA model could this be explained? One explanation would be if in fact women's best interests were not the Committee's dominant preference. We shall argue in due course for a view which could be mistaken for precisely this claim; so let us make clear why we are here rejecting it. We are assuming that on the RA model, the rational actor's preferences are *either* preferences which she has consciously formulated to herself (e.g. in arriving at an ordered ranking of them); *or* if she has not consciously formulated them to herself, they are ones which she would sincerely acknowledge as hers if they were put to her. But we are excluding from her range of preferences any factors which, although perhaps influencing her conduct, are ones which she has neither consciously entertained, nor would sincerely acknowledge as hers if the issue were put to her. (Such an unconscious, non-preference, action-directing factor might be, for example, an ideology of the kind envisaged by Marx, or possibly a Freudian unconscious wish.) So in accepting that the Committee's dominant preference was for the best practicable facilities in the area of breast cancer, we are rejecting any conspiracy theories. We are not supposing that the Committee were cynically pursuing something which they knew not to be in women's best interests.

So, is the assumption that they believed the screening programme to be the best available option something that the RA model would predict? We have implicitly begun to argue for a 'No' answer to this question in arguing that the evidence available to a rational enquiry would have revealed the flaws in the programme (the very flaws which were discussed in Chapter 2). Of course, if the Committee had been unaware of these flaws, then the RA account might still be the right explanation. But it is very implausible to think that the Committee *could* have been unaware of the flaws. Most of the Committee members were experts in the field, and the articles and research reports in which the evidence against the screening programme appeared were readily available. Further, although as we have noted, the Committee itself consisted only of those who were antecedently in favour of screening or were antecedently neutral, and contained no known critics of the screening programme, the Committee must have been aware of the weaknesses of the programme since they took evidence from consulting experts, a number of whom (such as Skrabanek, Ellman and Roberts) were vocal and severe critics.

It would still be possible to save an RA explanation of the Committee's decisions if we could assume that although the Committee was aware of the criticisms that had been made of the screening programme, they thought that these criticisms could somehow be met. But there is no evidence that the Committee did think this. The Report contains no discussion or rebuttal of the criticisms; and since (as was pointed out in Chapter 1 the minutes of all its meetings have now been destroyed, there is no evidence that the Committee had any reasoned objections to the prevalent criticisms. It seems that they heard the criticisms, were fully aware of them, and without knowing how to meet them, then simply expunged them from their minds when they came to make their recommendations. No pure RA model could explain such behaviour.

Recogising the deficiencies of a pure RA model when it is used to explain actual real-world choices, some theorists have proposed modified versions of the pure RA account which we were considering above. In the following two sections, two such accounts are examined, Simon's 'bounded rationality' account, and Lindblom's 'limited comparisons' account, to see if they are more successful than the pure version of the RA theory. Since some of the points which were made above will apply also to Simon and to Lindblom, our discussion of them can be more brief.

4 Simon's 'bounded rationality' model

Simon (1957) takes over from the RA model the thought that the behaviour of agents and organisations can at least sometimes be explained in rational terms; but he offers a different account of the deliberative processes which lead up to and explain the decision.

More specifically, what he retains is the idea that agents have an ordered set of preferences, and that they have information about the cost and benefits of various courses of action, and likelihoods of success in those actions bringing the satisfaction of the various preferences. So far, he sounds like an orthodox RA theorist. Where he differs from the 'pure' versions of RA theory which we considered above is in his account of the preferences of agents. On pure RA model, the rational agent, having worked out her ordered set of preferences, then investigates *all* the subgoals which those preferences generate; and then *all* the sub-sub-goals; and so on. And for each of these routes to a possible preference satisfaction, the rational actor works out the expected utility.

Simon insists that whether or not this complexity is required for an adequate account of 'rationality' in some sense of the term, it is psychologically implausible at best, psychologically impossible at worst. Agents simply do not have the capacity is engage in that kind of highly caculative manipulation of facts about themselves. Rather, what they do is simplify the problems that confront them by focusing on only a few possibilities, and making their choice from amongst them. For example, in deciding which university to apply to, a Simonian agent will not send away for prospectuses from *every* university (not even from every university *in the country!*). Rather, what she is likely to do is to select a relatively small number of universities to investigage in depth, and she will make her choice from them. And of course the crucial point here is that her selection of the relatively small number of universities which she is going to investigate is not made in the way that a pure RA model would predict. Rather, it can be made on a variety of 'irrational' grounds ('received wisdom', 'intuition', hearsay, etc.)

Already, Simon's account sounds psychologically more realistic than pure RA models. But how successful is it if we apply it to our test case, the decisions of the Forrest Committee? As in our discussion of the pure RA model, there are two ways in which we can test the theory. We can ask first, given the assumed information and ordered preferences of the Committee, what recommendations would the theory predict? Or secondly, we could again work backwards from the recommendations, and ask whether the information and preferences which the theory would then postulate are plausible ones to attribute to the Committee.

In relation to the first of these, our calculations can be very similar to those for the pure RA model. A Simonian account would attribute to the Committee a range of information perhaps rather narrower than that attributed by the RA model (i.e. it would postulate that the Committee would limit its attention 'non-rationally' to only *some* of the possible means of achieving the Committee's preferred goals). It thus predicts that the Committee would consider breast cancer screening as an option, along with the other sorts of possibilities which we have already mentioned (awaiting the results of the the UK survey, recommending further research on improving biopsy techniques, etc). And given the twin assumptions *both* that the screening programme was not in women's best interests, *and* that the Committee was aiming at women's best interests, the Simonian account would not predict that the Committee would make the recommendation that they did.

Suppose that we pursue the reverse route, and work back from the actual recommendations to an assumed range of information and set of preferences. The argument will then be very much as rehearsed in the previous section: there is no reason to think the Committee was engaged in a cynical conspiracy; there is no reason to think that they were unaware of the objections to screening; there is no evidence that they had any idea how to meet the objections. The existence of the objections seems simply to have been blotted from their minds when they made the recommendations. In other words, if we adopt the Simonian model,we cannot render consistent the Committee's recommendations with any set of preferences and aby body of informatio which we can plausibly assume they were acting on. And this implies that that Simonian model will not give us the adequate explanation which we are searching for.

5 Lindblom's 'limited options' model

Lindblom is another theorist who agrees with Simon that the model of the rational decision maker is generally implausible if taken as offering an explanation of how humans do actually make decisions. In Lindblom (1959), he maintains that the rational approach, or as he calls it the rational comprehensive model is impossible. His general criticism is that:

> It assumes intellectual capacities and sources of information that men simply do not possess, and it is even more absurd as an approach to policy when the time and money that can be

allocated to a policy problem is limited, as is always the case (Lindblom, 1959, p. 80)

For example, he says, it is very implausible to think that individuals engaged in decision-making have a consistent order of preferences, especially when those preferences include what we can loosely call matters of value. Commenting on his own 'preferences set', Lindblom remarks that he knows 'of no way to describe or even understand what my relative evaluations are for, say, freedom and security'. Again, he agrees with Simon that it is quite unrealistic to think that in practice, decision-makers try to take account of *all* the possible options which in theory confront them. In practice, they simply ignore a wide range of theoretically possible options and instead concentrate on only a few. Where he differs from Simon is in his account of what determines which options are taken seriously and explored. As we saw above, Simon thinks that the principle determinant is not so much rational assessment of evidence pro and con, but rather a kind of received (possibly folk) wisdom. Lindblom describes a process which he calls 'successive limited comparisons'. What this means is that in the selection of which options to take seriously, decision-makers do not start with (as it were) a blank sheet of paper and no pre-conceptions. They start from the existing state of affairs and consider only those courses of action which make small changes to the existing state of affairs. They do not in general ask the question whether the status quo is *totally* wrong. Rather, they take it as given, and ask how it can be improved.

Thus policy choice tends to focus on consideration of options which offer different marginal combinations of values. This means that the decision maker need not be involved in a deep analysis of all of the relevant values but rather only with those that differ from each other marginally. This tendency to concentrate on marginal differences coupled with the tendency of western democracies to change policies slowly and in a series of small steps means that 'policy does not move in leaps and bounds'.

Furthermore, Lindblom argues, it is not just the case that policy makers *do* limit the focus of their attention in this way; it is also (he claims) desirable that they should do so, because that is the only way of making effective use of available knowledge.

Given the limits on knowledge within which policy makers are confined, simplifying by limiting the focus to small variations from present policy makes the most of available knowledge (p. 92)

The strategy of considering only small incremental changes has

(Linblom believes) other advantages, in particular the fact that there is a smaller likelihood of making serious and lasting mistakes. For:

> In the first place, past sequences of policy steps have given [the decision-maker] knowledge about the probable consequences of further similar steps. Second he need not attempt big jumps towards his goals that would require predictions beyond his or anyone else's knowledge because he never expects his policy to be a final resolution of the problem. His decision is only one step, one that if successful can quickly be followed by another. Third, he is able to test his previous predictions as he moves to each further step. Lastly, he can often remedy a past error fairly quickly (p. 93)

What, then, is the result of applying Lindblom's 'limited options' theory of explanation to the Forrest Committee? Can it provide us with a satisfactory explanation of the decisions of the Committee? As when we were considering the RA model and Simon, let us ask first what recommendations we would expect the Committee to make, given the Lindblom theory.

Like Simon, Lindblom thinks that in general decision-makers will not in practice try to access huge amounts of potentially relevant information about the options they are considering. But in the case of something as specialised as breast cancer screening, it would not be unreasonable to assume that Lindblom's account would attribute to the Committee very much the same range of information as would be ascribed to it by both the RA and Simonian accounts. And given that the Committee was set up with the brief that it should examine the pros and cons of breast cancer screening, Lindblom would obviously include a cancer screening programme as *one* of options which the Committee would consider. But equally, given his expectation that policy changes in small incremental steps, his model would also predict that other options the Committee would consider would be those that made only marginal changes to the status quo. The most obvious of these would be one which we have mentioned before, namely awaiting the results of the UK trial. This would not have involved any large commitment of new resources by the Government, nor the setting up of new institutional structures. Other options which his model would predict that the Committee would consider include extending, for example, to improve the interpretation of mammograms, to make biopsies more senstive. As we have seen, these were known to be areas in which the screening programme was problematic. So a recommendation to improve techniques in these areas *before* the launch of a national screening programme (with all the attendant expense and commitment of adminstrative resources) would (in Lindblomian terms) be an obvious option for the Committee to consider.

But (and this is where his theory fails to give an adequate explanation), it is very surprising on his account that the Committee should have recommended the setting up of a national screening programme. For of all the options, this is the one which inolved the most radical break with the past, and is therefore the one which on Lindblom's theory would be the leat expected. Whatever the merits, then, of the Lindblom approach when applied to other examples, we conclude that it cannot give us a satisfactory account of the behaviour of the Forrest Committee.

6 Wildavsky's account

The final theorist whom we will consider, Aron Wildavsky, offers an interestingly different account of how appeals to ratinality function in the explanation of institutional decision-making. We shall shall argue in fact that Wildavsky is confused in the position which he seeks to defend, but that we can salvage something of interest from what he says, by reconstructing two different, and indeed incompatible, accounts.

On the first of these accounts, Wildavsky (let us call him Wildavsky I in this role) appears as a radical critic of all version of an RA model. His principal criticism focuses on the preferences (or goals, as he calls them) which rational actors are supposed to have. In places, he seems to think that the supposeldy rational agents, do not *have* an ordered set of preferences. Thus he asks:

> How can we be goal-directed if we don't know what our goal is until we get there? (Wildavsky 1979, p. 135).

And he quotes with approval Karl Weick's remark:

> It is difficult for a person to be rational if he does not know precisely what it is that he is supposed to be rational about (Wilavsky, 1979, p. 136)

The implication of the first of these quotation seems to be not that we do have [an ordered set of] goals, although we do not know what they are; but rather that we do not have such a set at all. Since, as we have seen in section two of this chapter, all RA models presuppose that the agents do have some ordered set of goals, Wildavsky I's denial of this would immediately destroy all possibility of an RA explanation of the behaviour of such social actors.

Wildavsky I does not, however, deny that RA language is widely used in the context of decision-making, nor that it has an important role to play in that context. What he insists is that that role is not an *explanatory* one. Rather, it is used (in his own word) to 'rationalise' behaviour after it has occurred. What he envisages is that once the action has occurred, the agents attribute to their past selves sets of goals (and implicitly bodies of information) in the light of which their action would have been the rational one to perform (rational according to RA theory). But these goals and data which agents attribute to themselves were not the *real explainers* of the action. It was not *because* the agent had those goals and data that she acted as she did. Indeed, the implication of Wildavsky I's position seems to be that the agent need not have had those goals and data at all for the attribution of them to be legitimate.

An alternative way of putting this point would be to distinguish between two senses of 'explanation'. If to explain something is merely to render it intelligible, then Wildavsky I allows that the use of RA models can explain behaviour. They enable the actors to *make sense of* their past actions, to fit them into *meaningful patterns*, and to discern a *coherent continuity* in what they have done. (We could call this post hoc explanation). But if to explain something means to identify the real factors which have brought it about, then Wildavsky I is clearly denying that RA models can yield explanation of real world decisions. (We could call this, perhaps rather tendentiously, real explanation).

That this is indeed Wildavksy I's position is confirmed when he says that the retrospective atribution of goals and data 'is done to increase the coherence of past actions' (p. 136), i.e. it is not done because it provides real explanations, in the sense of that term described above. He says that 'one acts first and makes sense of it *later*', and that we are engaged in 'attributing *new* motivational meaning to what we have done' (ibid). He refers to 'our ability to make what we have done conform to reason as we understand it *after we have acted*' (p. 137 - italics added in all three quotations). In short, Wildavsky I confines the role of RA language to an 'as if' level. After one has acted, one can interpret one's actions, both to others and to oneself, *as if* they were rational. In other words, one can give them a post hoc explanation. But although one's actions can be *in accord with* the dictates of rationality, it is not *because* they are in accord with those dictates that they are performed; and these rational considerations do not therefore supply the real explanation for the decision.

What, then, *is* the right explanatory model which we choose prefer to RA accounts? On this question, Wildavsky I is largely silent. All he tells us on this question is (in words which he quotes from Weick again) that:

> If we watch closely, it will become clear the behaviour [of social decision-makers] is under the control of more determinants that just the vocally stated plan [i.e. the plan that 'rational' decision-makers would produce] (ibid.)

But what these 'more determinants' are which actually produce and thereby explain the behaviour of the decision-makers, Wildavsky I does not describe. He summarises his overall scepticism about the usefulness of RA model by saying that in the field of social decision 'There is, in a word, a little rationality, though not a whole lot' (Wildavsky, 1979, p. 135)

Because Wildavsky I has so little of a positive kind to say about the real explanation, the further 'determinants' referred to above, we cannot usefully ask what explanation he would provide of the Forrest Committee's recommendations, nor seek to retrodict from their recommendations to the nature and content of any prior deliberations. We can, however, ask ourselves how plausible his claims are about the absence of a dominant goal which the Forrest Committee can be taken to have pursued.

On this issue, Wildavsky I is in one way implausible, and in another way plausible. He is implausible if he is taken to mean that the Committee was not aware at the time of its deliberations and recommendations that the provision of the best practicable facilities for breast cancer was its principal goal. How to achieve that goal was, after all, implicit in their terms of reference, and it was because of their expertise in that domain that the Committee members were selected, Forrest himself by the Government, and the remaining Committee members by Forrest. The idea, implicit in the first quotation above, that the Committee 'did not know what their goal was until they got there' sounds absurd.

But if what Wildavsky I means here is that in practice the Committee would have had other goals which they could not have ordered consistently, the criticism is probably true. We mentioned above in section 2 how it is implicit in the very idea of a committee of experts set up to issue recommendations that there are constraints on the time they can take for their deliberations, on the expenses they can occur, and so on. It is very unlikely that the Committee ever discussed the relative weighting to be attached to each of these aims — how they would rank in order of preference, for example, underspending their budget by 50% and being a day late with their Report, as against delivering the Report on time and overshooting the budget by 3%. Wildavsky I's point here is very much the one which we have seen that Simon and Lindblom in their different ways both insist on — RA decision-making in practice only takes place within a narrow range of options. Much that could in theory be considered, and from a pure RA point of view shouldbe considered, is simply taken for granted.

There is, however, a second and in some ways more interesting interpretation of Wildavsky (what we will call Wildavsky II). Wildavsky II is (unlike Wildavsky I) solidly within the RA tradition. Like Wildavsky I, he puts a question against the preferences which a 'commonsense' application of the RA model would assume. But whereas Wildavsky I doubts whether there are any preferences, or ordered sets of them, prior to the action, Wildavksy II *does* believe that actors have such preferences, that they do act on these preferences, and that these preferences can therefore supply real and not merely post hoc explanations. Where he differs from Wildavsky I (and from other RA theorists such as Simon and Lindblom) is in the preferences which he thinks actually move people to action. For the preferences which he postulates are (from a 'commonsense' perspective) very surprising.

This point is well illustrated by an example which Wildavsky quotes from environmental decision-making. The Delaware River was very heavily polluted, and the Delaware River Basin Commission sought, with the aid of expert committees etc, to formulate a policy for cleaning up the river. An immensely costly programme was set up, involving five states and costing hundreds of millions of dollars. In terms of cleaning up the estuary the programme was largely a failure. Pollution levels were lowered to some extent, but not by very much. And they could have been lowered to almost the same degree at a *very* much lower cost. Furthermore, these facts about relative costs and benefits were known *before* the decisions were taken. On the face of it, this looks to be a case of wild irrationality — of authorities deliberately choosing policies which they know will not maximise their expected utility.

But what Wildavsky does is to challenge the natural-seeming assumption that the dominant preference of those responsible for public choices in this area was a cost-efficient cleaning of the river. Rather, he says, the dominant preference was to be seen to be doing something *serious* about environmental pollution. From this point of view, the higher costs of some schemes over others was not a disutility, but in a strange kind of utility. It was a measure of how seriously one took the problem, of what sacrifices one was prepared to solve it, etc. Whether the policy was *actually* going to be the most efficient at cleaning the river became a side-issue. If we change in this way the preferences which we attribute to the actors, their decisions, far from seeming bizarrely irrational, can be seen as eminently rational. Their dominant preference was for a policy which would unambiguously proclaim their attachment to the importance of the environment, and that is exazctly the policy which was adopted. Wildavsky remarks of the very modest improvement in the cleanliness of the river that it is not much gain for approximately three quarter of a billion dollars, not much, that is, if you value results. But if the cleaning is what you value, if your aim is the ritual of purification, then the whole thing is a rip-roaring success (Wildavsky, 1979, p. 184)

What Wildavsky then seeks to do is to seek confirming evidence for the hypothesis that this 'ritual of purification' was indeed what the participants were aiming at. This evidence comes from examining the way in which the various participants did not wish to be 'upstaged' by rivals in the purification stakes.

How, then, can we apply Wildavsky II's ideas to the Forrest Committee's decisions? From the account given above, we can see that there must be two stages. First, we must abandon the assumption which we have been making so far that the Committee's dominant goal was the provision of the best practicable facilities for breast cancer, and postulate some other dominant preference in the light of which their decisions would have been rational. But secondly, if this postulation is not to be merely arbitrary, we would have to find independent confirming evidence that the Committee really was moved by such goals. If what we want is a real explanation and not just a post hoc one, we need to know not merely that their actions would have been rational if they had had those postulated preferences, but (more strongly) that they *did* have those preferences and were acting on them when they made the decisions they did.

Rather than address directly the question of how far Wildavsky II could provide a real explanation of the Forrest Committee's decisions, we want to turn aside to consider what may seem a side-issue. The justification for this is that if the argument which we are about to mount is correct, it will place severe constraints on the goals which Wildavsky II can postulate in his attempt to bring seemingly irrational behaviour within the ambit of the RA account. The question is one that was touched on earlier in section 3 above. It is this: on an RA account, how conscious does a person have to be of her preferences? There are a range of possible criteria here. A very demanding one would be that for an action to count as rational, the agent must *at the time* have been conscious of the preferences on which she was acting. This criterion is surely too restrictive. It would have the conseauence, for example, that many habitual actions could not count as rational. Yet surely if we calculate, in an approved RA manner, that a particular savings plan is the most rational one for me, we do not have to rehearse the calculations each month in order for monthly payments to count as rational. The original rational caculation can surely transfer its rationality to an idefinitely large number of other actions. A less demanding criterion would say that *at some point in the past*, we must consciously have rehearsed our list of goals if the action is to be rational. This more liberal criterion would allow that each of the monthly payments can count as rational even though on none of them are we consciously thinking about maximising expected utilities. But perhaps even this criterion is too restrictive. It may be that a person can properly be said to have dominant preference in a particular area, even if at no time has she consciously formulated it to herself. Evidence that she did nevertheless have thar preference would come from her behaviour, both verbal and non-verbal. Verbally, if challenged as to whether she had that preference, she would be willing to acknowledge it; non-verbally, the assumption that she had that preference would enable us to make sense of a wide variety of her actions.

Once we envisage countenancing preferences which move beyond this third and most undemanding of criteria, we are envisaging 'preferences' which the agent has never consciously entertained, and which she would not acknowledge as her own if they were put to her. She might even vigorously and sincerely deny that she had them. But if factors as distant as this from the actor's caculations about what to do are allowed to count as genuine *preferences* in an RA model, then we have lost all sense of a contrast between explanatory theories like the RA accounts on the one hand, and those (like, for example Marxist ideological explanations) which invoke non-conscious but functional determinants of action.

It is in order to meet this problem that it is *essential* to

Wildavsky II's project that he should be able to find the extra confirming evidence referred to in the second step outlined three paragraphs above. In the absence of that second step, the factors which might be invoked as instances of an agent's goals or preferences could all fail to meet even the most liberal of our three criteria above for being a genuine preference/goal. The upshot is that whatever factors a Wildavsky II explanatin for Forrest might postulate would have to be factors which, at the very least, the Committee would itself have been willing to acknowledge. To show conclusively that there are no such factors would be a very large undertaking (it is an instance of the general problem of proving the non-existence of something), and it is not one which will be explicitly tackled here. What we will do instead in subsequent chapters is to identify what we take to be the most likely candidates for these non-conscious determinants of the Committee's actions, and show that they fit much better into a quite different account of explanation from the one Wildavsky II proposes, and that there is thus no need to try to force them into an RA straightjacket.

We have so far spent a good deal of time looking at possible explanations provided by the RA model and its variants. Although the verdict has in the end been unfavourable to these types of explanation, this emphasis has been an entirely natural one. The RA family of models contains some appealing ideas, and even one of its critics has observed of it that:

> it generates subtle, elegant and powerful theorems from very simple assumptions (Hollis, 1987, p. 15)

and again, Hollis writes:

> The theory of rational choice does a precise job very neatly. It . . . gives economics a starting point. If 'choice' is extended to any allocation of resources, itmay perhaps do the same for our understanding of social action at large. That makes it a hugely interesting theory (p.26)

There are, indeed, other variants of the RA model which we could consider, such as those provided by Etzioni (1967), Hogwood and Gunn (1984), or Bender and Moe (1985). But rather than pursue these variants of the RA accounts, we now to turn to a theory of a rather different kind, one which (we will argue) is more promising than any which we have so far examined.

71

7 Sabatier's account

Sabatier starts his account by focusing on the link between values and beliefs, and on their role in policy making (Sabatier, 1988). There are clearly some similarities between Sabatiers' approach and that of Lindblom and Simon, in that they also imagine that the guiding principle behind the choice of policy options is a hierarchy of values. With this, Sabatier has no quarrel since he also thinks that what motivates policy makers is their desire to transform their values and beliefs into policy.

Sabatier accepts Heclo's assertion (Heclo, 1981) that within any given area there will be individuals (and groups) who are in conflict with each other. But he adds two further ideas to this starting point. First, he claims that policy-making can be conceptualised in the same way as belief systems, i.e. as 'sets of value priorities and causal assumptions about how to realise them' (Sabatier,1988). Secondly, he claims that there is no single or specific governmental institution which would provide a useful focus for the study of policy- making (Sabatier,1988). Rather, it is more useful to look at *policy sub-systems*, each of which includes a wide variety of actors who all involved in the formation of policy in that specific area.

A policy sub-system, according to Sabatier, does not consist simply of a small number of 'experts', since a wide variety of actors play an important role in the dissemination of ideas and information. The concept of such a sub-system therefore needs to cover journalists, researchers and interest groups, as well as those individuals involved in policy formation at a lower level within the governmental hierarchy. He defines a policy sub-system as a group of individuals who are closely concerned with a policy area. Sabatier also points out that although it is essential to include in any analysis of policy subsystems those individuals who are active, it is also importnat to identify latent actors, as they might become active at some point in the future and prove critical in changing the balance of power within a given policy sub-system.

It would, however, be a mistake Sabatier maintains to think that members of a policy sub-system form a single homogeneous group. Within a policy subsystem, so-called 'advocacy coalitions' emerge. These are collections of individuals who share a set of normative beliefs, and who form groups in order to further policy objectives. In most policy subsystems, the number of advocacy coalitions is likely to be small. (For example, in discussing the debate about air pollution in the USA, Sabatier distinguishes twelve advocacy coalitions). This is because in order achieve the desired policy outcome, small groups tend to coalesce with the larger ones in order to increase their strength. Two aspects of these advocacy coalitions are of particular note: first, the system of beliefs which is shared by all members of a given coalition; and secondly, the role of such coalitions in promoting policy-oriented learning. We will comment on each of the aspects.

The shared belief system provides what might be called the 'glue' of politics. In analysing such belief systems, he distinguishes three levels at which beliefs may be held: deep core, near core, and secondary aspects. Deep core beliefs are a person's 'fundamental normative and ontological axioms'. In other words, the deep core consists of a person's most deeply held values. They are a fundamental part of the individual's normative framework, and they are highly resistant to change. Near core beliefs concern policy objectives; and although they are resistant to change, they are not as resistant as deep core beliefs. Secondary aspects consist of a variety of instrumental beliefs about what causes what. They therefore concern the way in which policies should be implemented. Since these beliefs are highly instrumental, they are relatively open to change. To give an example of these three levels: a person might hold to freedom of information as one of her deep core beliefs; this might be associated with the near core policy of supporting e.g. a freedom of information act; while the secondary aspects would cover the detailed tactics necessary to get such an act onto the statute book.

The second important aspect of advocacy coalitions is their role in promoting policy-oriented learning. Like Heclo, Sabatier sees these groups as being in conflict with each other, a conflict which is mediated by individuals (or groups) whom he calls policy brokers. The policy learning which Sabatier is here referring to arises as a result of the argument and debate between the conflicting groups. These debates will characteristically be conducted by experts who are in touch with current research findings in the relevant field. This is not to say that the groups are entirely open-minded and unbiased in their debates with each other. Indeed, as new knowledge emerges within any given policy area, groups will use it in highly partisan ways. If any new knowledge or information emerges which conflicts with their existing beliefs, it may well be ignored.

This policy-oriented learning can occur in various domains. Sabatier picks out three areas for especial notice. There is firstly the task of improving understanding, and keeping up to date with changes and innovations which directly affect the belief systems. Secondly, learning can be about improving one's understanding of causal relationships internal to one's belief systems. This would

73

involve the search for new mechanisms through which the policy objective might be more easily and effectively achieved. Thirdly, there is responding to challenges to one's belief system.

But Sabatier does not think that policy-oriented learning is the only factor which effects policy change over time. Another important influence is the socio-economic climate. He argues that although policy-oriented learning is important when considering policy changes over time, changes in the *core* aspects of a policy are usually the results of perturbations in the 'non-cognitive factors external to the sub-system', such as macro-economic conditions. He makes a distinction between two different types of perturbations. There are, first, those which he calls 'dynamic system events'. These are events which have a good chance of changing belief systems or of encouraging policy-oriented learning. Secondly, there are changes to the 'relatively stable parameters' which most political systems display.

Although members of different advocacy coalitions may be separated by major differences in their core beliefs, constructive dialogue can nevertheless occur between them. In order for such dialogue to take place, both sides must first have both the incentive and the resources to engage in such a debate. Secondly, they must have sufficient technical resources to be able to criticise each others' claims, for example, about what are the relevant data, what causal mechanisms achieve what results, etc. Furthermore, the debate is likely to be most productive if it centres on differences between the secondary aspects of the two belief systems, since an all-out attack on each others' core belief is likely to produce no more than defensive reactions.

In order to illustrate the structure and interactions of belief systems and policy orientation, Sabatier uses the example of two pressure groups which were involved in the debate about air pollution in the USA: the Clean Air Coalition, and the Economic Efficiency Coalition. These two groups had been fundamentally divided over the extent to which the pursuit of individual freedom in a market economy should be constrained in order to protect the health of 'susceptible populations' (e.g. those already suffering from respiratory diseases). Members of the Clean Air Coalition argued that the protection accorded to the susceptible populations to be absolute, while the members of the Economic Efficiency Coalition have been more willing to put them at risk in the interests of individual liberty and increased production. This normative difference in the policy core of the two coalitions probably reflected a deep core difference in the relative priority accorded freedom (or efficiency) versus equality, a conflict underlying many policy disputes (Sabatier, 1988, p. 135)

This extract highlights the way in which advocacy coalitions can come into conflict with each other, and the way that such conflicts often reveal differences in the deep core belief system.

In the debate about air pollution in the USA, it may appear that the two advocacy coalitions were roughly equal in size and power. But Sabatier maintains that within any given policy sub-system there is likely to be a dominant advocacy coalition, and while this advocacy coalition remains dominant the basic attributes of government policy are unlikely to change significantly. It follows from this that a minority advocacy coalition has little hope of changing its place within the sub-system or of effecting policy.

Sabatier, then, sees the role of policy-oriented learning as being crucial in the development of policy over time; not because the conflict between the groups gradually decreases as they tend towards consensus, but because policy becomes better informed as time goes on. Unlike previous writers, he tends not to focus on a straightforward notion of rationality (or lack of it), but rather he looks at the role played by the belief systems of those involved in the 'game' of politics. Although this approach offers an interesting alternative to previous ones, it is not without its difficulties.

8 An assessment of Sabatier

A first doubt that could be raised about Sabatier's account is whether he is correct in his assumption that it is learning, or in particular, policy-oriented learning, that influences policy change. At one point, Sabatier remarks that:

> Policy oriented learning refers to relatively enduring alterations of thought or behavioural intentions which result from experience and which are concerned with the attainment (or revision) of policy objectives (Sabatier, 1988, p. 133).

This description of learning implies that the kind of learning that occurs within the policy-making arena is exactly the same learning that occurs elsewhere, or at least that it covers every (rational) change in thought. That is to say that it:

1 Requires long-term alteration of thought or intentions
2 Is caused by experience
3 Is concerned with policy objectives.

If this is the case, then it is hard to see why Sabatier draws a distinction between policy-oriented learning on the one hand, and 'non-cognitive factors external to the sub-system' on the other; for both of these 'cause' policy- oriented learning, by Sabatiers' (1988) definition of that phrase. Anyway, it is difficult to see where 'external events' do not entail learning. Perhaps it would be more useful to put it thus: policy-oriented learning is that learning which explains changes in secondary aspects of a belief system. But then it is not clear whether that would include the deep core and the near core. It would seem unlikely that real world changes would have much effect on deep core values as he describes them. For example, it is difficult to see how the oil boycott could effect an individual's view on whether human beings are evil or not.

This brings us to a second difficulty with Sabatier's model, a difficulty concerning the structure of the belief systems. Before outlining the threefold structure of belief systems, Sabatier points to three important features of the actors involved in policy-making. Firstly, the actors wish to maximise their utility and are rational in the choices by which they try to realise that aim. However, Sabatier thinks that group wants and goals can be given more weight than individual goals. Secondly, there is an assumption of 'limited rationality'. And thirdly, policy sub-systems are composed of policy elites, who will have belief systems which are both complex and internally consistent. (Rational choices/goals based on non-cognitive core beliefs?)

Sabatier then describes the three categories into which he says that beliefs can be placed. But there are several problems with this framework. Firstly, Sabatier does not justify the assumption that beliefs should be, or can be, placed into three categories in terms of their resistance to change. If the crucial variable is resistance to change, why not say two categories, or four, or any other number? Sabatier supplies no good theoretical justification for his preference for a tripartite division. It is is surely more accurate to say simply that individuals have a set of beliefs, some of which are more resistant to change than others. They can no doubt be ranged on a spectrum, running from those that are very resistant to change all through to those that are highly provisional. But the idea that they fall naturally into three classes is unwarranted.

Further, even if we grant that the threefold division in terms of degree of resistance to change is useful, there is no good reason for associating with each category, beliefs that have a particular content. Why, for example, should normative beliefs occur only in the deep core? Why could a person not hold some of her normative beliefs in a tentative way, hence in a way that was relatively open to change, and hence in a way that is characteristic of Sabatier's secondary aspects? For example, a person might hold the normative belief that torture is always wrong, and hold this belief in a highly entrenched, 'deep core' way. But another normative belief (e.g. that euthanasia is sometimes morally permissible) might be one that she held only provisionally, and it would therefore be quite open to change. Equally, why should not some empirical means-end beliefs be very highly confirmed, hence very resistant to change, and hence located in Sabatier's deep core? An individual might hold the means/end belief that other things being equally, increasing the cost of an item will reduce effective demand for it. But even if this belief is very highly entrenched, and hence a prime candidate for Sabatier's deep core, there is nothing normative about it.

But there are also further criticisms to be made of Sabatier's use of the concept of deep core beliefs. One initial question is how deep core beliefs can be identified in the first place. Sabatier's own suggestion is:

> to allow actors to indicate their belief systems (via questionnaires and content analysis of documents) and then empirically examine the extent to which these change over time (p. 124).

But this suggestion is unpromising. In the first place, it is a very naive approach to discovering what people's belief systems are. Secondly, there is a problem associated with the kinds of sources he mentions. Discovering an individual's belief system is difficult enough. Even if individuals are willing to complete questionnaires designed to find out what their deep core beliefs are, there is still the problem that an individual may not be clear what her deep core beliefs are. And even when she is sure in her own mind what they are, there may be the further difficulty of finding an adequate articulation for them. The identification of the individual's core beliefs may thus depend on interpretation and inference by the researcher, and this introduces a further element of uncertainty into the exercsie. How much more difficult, then, would it be to discover the core beliefs of an advocacy coalition, let alone of an entire policy sub-system.

There is, then, a problem about the identificaton of the core beliefs. But even if we assume that this problem can be overcome, Sabatier's claim that advocacy coalitions will be united by shared core beliefs is implausible. Agents who are allies within a particular advocacy coalition might have few if any shared deep core beliefs at all. Some coalitions might include very unlikely bedfellows. For example, Fascists may find themselves in a coalition with liberals over the issue of free speech. These two groups would certainly not share deep core values. Lindblom provides us with another example of the same phenomenon:

> It has been suggested that continuing agreement in Congress on the desirability of extending old-age insurance stems from the Liberal desires to strengthen the welfare programmes of the federal government and from conservative desires to reduce union demands for private pension plans. If so, this is an excellent demonstration of the ease with which individuals of different ideologies often can agree on concrete policy (Lindblom, 1959, p. 97).

Sabatier then goes on to a discussion of the relationships between interests and beliefs, and he claims that:

> This set of interests/goals, perceived causal relationships and perceived parameter states constitutes a 'belief system'. While belief system models can thus incorporate self/organisational interests, they also allow actors to establish goals in quite different ways (e.g. as a result of socialisation) and are therefore more inclusive (Sabatier, 1988, p. 161).

The thought here is, that 'interests' are a kind of 'special case' or 'sub-case' of belief systems. Sabatier sees interests and beliefs as being very closely linked. He claims that interest-based models have two elements, namely, (a) an accurate perception of 'real' interests, and (b) a knowledge of causal relationships (i.e. what to do to achieve what is really in your interests). Similarly, the belief system model also has two elements, namely (a) wants, and (b) a knowledge of causal relationships. The advantage of this second model, according to Sabatier, largely derives from the weaknesses of the first. The principal weakness focuses on how individuals can accurately identify what their 'real' interests are. Even in those cases in which they can confidently articulate a veiw about what their real interests are, they may well be wrong.

Sabatier's solution to this dilemma is that actors might well be more able to identify clearly and articulate what their beliefs are, and that furthermore, these are more easily verifiable and more open to investigation than are their supposed real interests. The problems associated with this have been mentioned earlier but there is a further difficulty. If, for the moment, we accept Sabatier's threefold division between deep core, near core and secondary aspects, then it would seem that the researcher would have very similar problems with respect to the slippery nature of core beliefs.

One final criticism of Sabatier concerns his account of how policy develop and become refined over time. As we have seen, he believes that this is a concsequence of the policy-oriented learning, which itself arises from coflicts between the various advocacy coalitions within a policy subsystem. Sabatier, and also to some extent the earlier rationality theorists, have all tended to ignore the role of the production of objective information which all of the models require if they are to function properly. Sabatier, like the other theorists, would concede that once the knowledge is available in the public arena, then it can be used in a highly instrumental way by policy makers. But the actual production of the objective information is not questioned. Since this seems to be of central importance to all of the models, it will be useful to consider briefly how information or evidence is produced.

Kuhn has already challenged the common belief that scientific knowledge is objective and value-free. Kuhn argues that during a period of so-called 'normal science', that new evidence and new theories which challenge the prevailing paradigm are resisted by the scientific community for as long as possible. Since even what counts as *evidence* can be partly determined by the prevailing paradigm, dominant groups within the scientific community can use various strategies to discount the supposed evidence of other groups. Martin (1979) lists the following manoeuvres used by scientists when they are faced with data which does not fit into the prevailing paradigm:

1 Flat denial
2 Scepticism about the source of the item
3 Ascription of an ulterior motive to the source
4 Isolation of the item
5 Minimalisation of the importance of the item
6 Interpretation of the item to suit one's purposes
7 Misunderstanding of the item, and
8 'Thinking away' or just forgetting the item.

Furthermore, it has been suggested that the process of debate and exchange of knowledge within an arena (Sabatier's example of such an arena is the field of professional journals, which is both high status and dominated by professional norms), does not necessarily facilitate the growth of learning. Rather, it serves to reinforce the values and beliefs of the dominant group or groups.

The process by which this occurs has been called the Gold Effect, (Gold, 1979) named after the man who first described the sequence of events: at the beginning a few people arrive at a state of near-belief in some idea. A meeting is held to discuss the pros and cons of the idea. More people favouring the idea than those who are uninterested or hostile will attend. A representative committee will be nominated to prepare a collective volume to propagate and foster interest in the idea. The totality of the resulting articles based on the idea will appear to show an increasing consensus. A specialised journal will be launched. Only orthodox or near-orthodox articles will pass the referees and the editor. The club of believers refuse to enter into discussion with their detractors, who are generally deemed to be irrational or professionally incompetent. The effect of all this is further accelerated by a glut of publications 'confirming' the idea, since young researchers eager for publication are encouraged to submit papers which align themselves to the accepted dogma.

The Gold Effect has been particularly noticeable in consensus statements, such as those regarding the role of diet on ischaemic heart disease. Such arenas therefore, according to Gold, have exactly the opposite effect to the one suggested by Sabatier, and do not engage in open and objective exchange of information.

9 The bureaucratic politics model

So far, a number of approaches have been considered to the question of how and why decisions are made, and all (or nearly all) of these approaches have focused on the rationality (or lack of it) of individual actors or groups within the policy-making arena. But an alternative theory which does not share this focus on rationality is supplied by the bureaucratic politics model. This move is important because it brings into focus the importance of *structures* within the decision making arena, in a way which almost disregards entirely the role played by beliefs in the way that Sabatier would suggest. Thus the two approaches (beliefs versus structures) represent two important aspects of the process that will be examined in some detail in chapter four.

The bureaucratic model suggests that policy emerges not as a rational choice by a central actor but as a result of bargaining between key personnel within the policy-making arena. Thus within government the various bureaucracies are represented by these individuals who bargain, propose or oppose various policies in terms of their bureaucratic interests. The government is therefore constituted by a whole range of competing groups who are all seeking to promote their own interests. This model focuses attention on the role of civil servants and their relationship to politicians.

Aberbach et al. (1981) outline four 'images' of this relationship:

Image One: This image presents perhaps the most idealistic notion of this relationship. It claims that politicians make policies and bureaucrats implement them. But however attractive this image might be, it is (as Aberbach et al. argue) an unlikely one. Solutions to even the most technical-seeming of problems can have policy implications, and the distinction between the political and the administrative is therefore ultimately untenable.

Image Two: The second image assumes, more realistically, that both politicians and bureaucrats take part in making policy. But it maintains the policy/administration distinction by claiming that politicians and civil servants make different contributions to the process of policy-making. Civil servants bring facts and knowledge while politicians bring interests and values.

Image Three: The third image recognises that both politicians and civil servants take part in making policy, and further that both are concerned with politics. The difference between them lies, as with the second image, in terms of their different contributions. But, unlike the account provided by the second image, the third image sees both groups as involved in advocating interests. The difference is only that (in Aberbach's words):

'whereas politicians articulate broad diffuse interests of organised individuals, bureaucrats mediate the narrow focused interests of organised clienteles' (1981 p.59).

The other important aspect of this image is that the system tends to have a bias against making radical change.

Image Four - In this final image, Aberbach tentatively suggests that the distinction drawn in the first three images between the politician and the bureaucrat is becoming so blurred that we are left with what he describes as a 'pure hybrid'.

But whether the bureaucrat is supposed to make political decisions the fact remains that they can and do. Within the model of bureaucratic politics, attention tends to be focused on processes and the possible effect they may have on policy. Heclo and Wildavsky (1981) examine the way the Treasury conducts its business. The picture that emerges corresponds very closely to the 'Yes Minister' atmosphere, where 'smooth as alabaster' figures like Sir Humphrey make all the important decisions through a process which seems to involve a combination of manipulation and polite bargaining. All of this is carried out between individuals who are very well-known to each other. 'The Chat' is the primary method of communication. Heclo and Wildavsky quote one Treasury assistant who comments:

> It is difficult for an outsider to appreciate how chummy things are in the civil service. You've probably known each other for fifteen years — lots of informal contact and socialising (Heclo and Wildavsky, 1981, p. 252).

They note that:

> Lunch can be taken within 500 yards at one of the clubs in Pall Mall, or even more convenient still at the Cabinet Office Mess, where ministers do not come. Membership is by invitation only, and attendance is a sign of acceptance into the upper reaches of the civil service (1981. p. 72).

Heclo and Wildavsky also cooment on the eixstence of a bias away from radical change. They note that individuals who enter the Treasury find it confusing initially. But then they gradually fit in as they discover that the major method of operating is 'the chat' and the interdepartmental contacts that have been built up over the years. If we could apply the 'images' described by Aberbach to Heclo and Wildavsky's study of the Treasury, then image three would probably be the closest, in that the civil servants certainly do serve the interests of a small clientele. The civil servants themselves do see a distinction between their roles and the roles of the ministers. Certainly a good Treasury man is in possession of knowledge and skills that the average minister does not have. But Heclo and Wildavsky do not believe that this necessarily leads to an unhealthy bias towards particular kinds of policy, except that it tends to be incremental.

So, the general premise of the bureaucratic politics model is that policy is a result of the bargaining between government departments who act largely in their own interests, this approach is well summed up in the old adage 'where you stand depends upon where you sit'. But this does not mean that bureaucrats are never innovative and never have ideas, and one of the common criticisms of this model is that it emphasises the role of interests too much and plays down the role of ideas.

Peters (1988) is one who denies that ideas have no important role to play. After making a distinction between 'hard' and 'soft' ideologies, and acknowledging that there is something called the 'departmental view', he challenges the notion that the Civil Service does not innovate. He argues that ideas within the Civil Service arise from two primary sources. Firstly, civil servants themselves often have a number of professional contacts, and they may use new ideas gained from such contacts to challenge existing policies. Secondly, increasing numbers of civil servants themselves have professional qualifications, or some form of professional training, and this expertise can be source of new ideas in debates about policy and its implementation. As examples of this sort of informed policy input by members of the bureaucracy, Peters instances both the movement for Medicare, and thedevelopment of community health programmes in the U.S.A.

Although writers interested in bureaucratic politics have tended to concentrate on the 'pulling and heaving' of politics, it is clear that ideas and ideology do have a role to play in the formation of policy and the functioning of departments. But whether these ideas are a result of intellectual brilliance, rational decision or the pursuit of interests is an intriguing question that to some extent remains unanswered.

10 Conclusion

Although many of the above theorists may disagree in certain areas, one thing that unites most of them is the premise that whatever policy options are being considered, some objective information is necessary in order for the policy makers to make a policy choice. In the case of breast cancer screening, it would be assumed that such information should be reliable empirical evidence; perhaps the implementation of Forrest was a result of this process? As was discussed earlier, the evidence for the effectiveness of breast cancer screening is far from conclusive. It could therefore be argued that the various types of rationality models fail adequately to explain the decisions of the Forrest Committee.

Comprehensive Rationality models, as with Lindblom's suggestion of an ideal type, would require the policy makers to consider all the information available from the randomised controlled trials. But as mentioned earlier, the Forrest Committee chose to consider a limited number of controlled trials as 'evidence'. Even when this approach is regarded as an example of the type of 'limited rationality' suggested by Simon, the processes by which some evidence was discarded while other pieces were retained remains difficult to explain.

The various 'cost-benefit' theories are also problematic since there was clear evidence to suggest that Breast Cancer Screening (even on the scale recommended by the Forrest Committee) would be a costly exercise, with the 'benefits' remaining difficult to define and difficult to predict.

The approach offered by the bureaucratic politics model initially looks more promising since clearly there were some gains in terms of resourcing for certain groups. Radiology departments, for example, expanded considerably in breast screening centres in order to cope with the increased workload. But as far as benefits for Whitehall departments is concerned, what few benefit there were, would not satisfactorily explain the decision to implement breast cancer screening.

The Sabatier model, which considers the role played by beliefs seems the most promising of all since it suggests that what motivates actors in the arena of politics is not short- term interests or even simple 'rationality' but deeply-held beliefs and values. Another advantage of the Sabatier style approach is that it can help to understand apparently 'irrational' decisions, especially if we consider Wildavskys' suggestion that what counts as 'rational' may actually not be as straightforward as at first thought. However, as has already been mentioned, Sabatier's approach faces a number of problems. In the following chapter, we will be considering a feminist reconstruction of the model offered by Sabatier, which will go some way to breaching the gaps in the model, and will produce a unique approach to the problem of analyzing the decision- making process.

References

Aberbach, J., Putnam, R., and Rockman, B; (1981), *Bureaucrats and Politicians in Western Democracies*, Harvard University Press, Cambridge, Mass.

Braybrooke, D., Lindblom, C; (1983); *A Strategy of Decision*, Free Press, New York.

Etzioni, A; (1967); 'Mixed Scanning: A Third Approach To Decision Making', *Public Administration Review*, Vol 27, pp. 385-392.

Gold, T; (1979); *Lying Truths: A Critical Scrutiny of Current Beliefs* and Conventions; Duncan, R., Weston-Smith, M., (eds), Pergamon Press, Oxford.

Greenaway, J., Smith, S., Street, J; (1992); *Deciding Factors In British Politics*, Routledge, London.

Heclo, H., Wildavski, A; (1981); *The Private Government of Public Money*, Macmillan Press, London.

Hogwood, B., Gunn, Lewis; (1984); *Policy Analysis For The Real World*, Oxford University Press, Oxford.

Hogwood, B; (1987); *From Crisis To Complacency?*, Oxford University Press, Oxford.

Hollis, M; (1983); *The Cunning of Reason*, Cambridge University Press, Cambridge.

Jenkins, B., Gary, A; (1983); 'Bureaucratic Politics and Power: Developments in the Study of Bureaucracy', *Political Studies* vol 135, pp. 177-193.

Lindblom, C; (1959); 'The Science of Muddling Through' *Public Administration Review* vol 19, pp. 78-99.

Lindblom, C; (1980); *The Policy Making Process*, Prentice Hall International, Englewood Cliffs, New Jersey.

Majone, G; (1975); 'The Feasibility of Social Policies', *Policy Sciences*, vol 6, pp. 49-69.

Marshall, N; (1986); 'Implementing Policy: A Bureaucratic Power Perspective', *The Australian Journal of Public Administration*, vol 1XLV, no1, pp. 18-29.

Marshall, N; (1988); 'The Failure of the Academic Lobby: from Policy Community to Bureaucratic Management', *Politics*, no 23, vol 2, pp. 67-79.

Martin, B; (1979); *Bis of Science*; Society for Social Responsibility in Science, Canberra, Australia.

Peters, G; (1988); *The Politics of Bureaucracy*, Longman, New York.

Sabatier, P; (1987); 'Top Down and Bottom up Approaches to Implementation Research: A Critical Analysis and Suggested Synthesis', *The Journal of Public Policy*, vol 6, no 1, pp. 21-48.

Sabatier, P; (1988); 'An Adversary Coalition Framework of Policy Change and the Role of Policy Oriented Learning Therein', *Policy Sciences*, vol 2, pp. 129-68.

Simon, H; (1957); *Administrative Behaviour*, MacMillan Press, New York.

Wass, D., (1984); *Government and the Governed*, Routledge and Keegan Paul, London.

Wildavsky, A; (1979); *The Art And Craft of Policy Analysis*, MacMillan Press, London.

Wildavsky, A and Heclo, H; (1981); *The Private Government of Public Money* Macmillan Press, London.

4 A feminist model of explanation

1 Introduction

The previous chapter was concerned with examining mainstream (male-stream) thinking about and models of decision- making. Of the various models discussed, the one suggested by Sabatier in his article 'An Advocacy Coalition Framework of Policy Change and the Role of Policy Oriented Learning Therein' is the most persuasive. Its particular strength lies in its concern with and acknowledgement of the roles played by beliefs in the process of policy-making and change. As we have already seen, there are problems associated with all the rational action models. Even the more cynical adaptations, such as the Lindblomian approach which suggests that policy-making is 'rational' only at the margins, are flawed. The alternative interest-based models often fail to connect interests and beliefs at all, even though, as Sabatier points out, interests and beliefs are inextricably bound up with one another. Sabatier really makes what in retrospect appears to be a rather obvious point, which is that human beings tend to act in accordance with their beliefs (even if these beliefs are not explicitly stated) and this is just as true in the world of policy-making as it is in any other area of life.

The principal concern here is with the weaknesses of Sabatier's model. As we saw in the previous chapter, none of the models considered provided us with a completely satisfactory theoretical understanding of the decsion making processess connected with the breast cancer screening programme. In this chapter we will be addressing these deficiencies. In particular, we will provide in this chapter a two-pronged critique of his theory. We will argue first, that the model does not consider the role of patriarchy; and secondly that the model gives insufficient consideration to the effect of power. These two areas can conveniently be labelled the areas of 'belief' and 'power'. It could be objected that these two areas are really a single indissoluble unit, since the concept of patriarchy must include not only a set of beliefs and values, but also a recognition of power relationships (e.g. those between men and women). But even if in practice patriarchy and power relationships always go hand in hand, we wish to keep the two concepts separate (initially at least) for theoretical purposes. Furthermore, these two concepts (of power and belief) need to be developed further in order that the ways in which they work within the policy making process is to be clearly understood and explained by the modification of Sabatier's model of decision making. These are vital elements within the process of political decision making for two reasons. Firstly, whatever model of decision making is considered, the process of negotiation and conflict, that is the meat and drink of policy making always occurs within a power structure. This power structure may be viewed in different ways by different commentators, but none would deny that it exists. Having accepted that a power structure exists, then its exact nature becomes of crucial importance. Especially since one of the main thrusts of this thesis is that the power structure is patriarchal in its nature. Secondly, a further development of the concept of beliefs is important because it needs to be clear that (a) patriarchal beliefs exist and that they have particular qualities, and (b) that the proposition that members of political elites possess them is a plausible claim.

What is envisaged, then, is a feminist reconstruction of Sabatier's model of decision-making, which incorporates the concepts of patriarchy and of power, giving them a significant role in the process of policy-making and change. We will first outline the need for a feminist dimension in general on the process of policy formation (section 2). Next, we will focus on patriarchy in sections 3 and 4, introduce the concept of power in section 5, and then consider them in combination in sections 6 and 7.

2 The need for a feminist dimension

Feminist writers have long been interested in the *effects* of public policies on the lives and welfare of women, especially since many of the decisions taken at the level of public policy affect mainly women. This is true, for example, in such areas as abortion, family and welfare policy, sex discrimination policies, etc. How the implementation of public policy affects women has therefore been the subject of much feminist debate. But what has not been the focus of any of these studies is the prior process of decision-making itself. Current analyses of the process of policy-making and policy-change do not consider whether the male-dominated nature of the world of politics (or indeed the male-dominated nature of the world of political scientists) has any important consequences in terms of policy outputs for the field of academic enquiry.

Lovenduski claims that this 'blindness' means that the models so far devised and the studies undertaken are completely inadequate:

> The complication here is that there never was any way that the modern study of politics could fail to be sexist. Its empirical concerns have been almost exclusively those of the exercise of public power, aspects of political elites and aspects of institutions of government. Such studies are bound to exclude women, largely because women usually do not dispose of public power, belong to political elites or hold influential positions in government institutions. In an increasingly positivistic discipline, no one thought to question this. The only enquiries in which women were scrutinised were empirical studies of the various components of political participation and predictably these studies contained numerous examples of sexist bias (Lovenduski, 1989, p. 89)

Lovenduski is referring us to the fact that the *structures* which political scientists examine are overwhelmingly dominated by men, that it is men who hold and dispose of public power, and that the vast majority of those academics involved in the study of these structures are also male, who have apparently failed to notice that women are 'not there'.

In order to correct this imbalance, it is necessary to develop a theory or model of decision-making which is not 'blind' to these issues. Such a model must begin by appreciating certain characteristics of the policy-making community and the policy-making process. In particular, three facts needed to be acknowledged.

First, given the almost total physical exclusion of women from the decision-making realm, it is clear that women are not controlling or disposing any significant degree of public power. We can concede that it is never the case that all the participants in the decision-making process are completely equal in power. But even given that some inequality is unavoidable, the massive under-representation of women is particularly striking, especially when it occurs in areas which primarily concern women and their interests.

Secondly, as far as the equal consideration of all knowledge is concerned, Lindblom has already shown that it is not humanly possible to consider every piece of evidence and every source of information relevant to an issue, and we would not argue with this. But the implication of this is that one must then accept that some *selection* takes place, a selection which determines which knowledge and which bits of information are counted as knowledge or information in the first place, and hence are given serious conside-ration. The prevalence of patriarchal beliefs, and the power relation-ships which flow from those beliefs, mean that women's knowledge and reasoning is often regarded as second-rate, and is hence largely ignored when important decisions are being taken.

Thirdly, given the overwhelming preponderance of men in the policy-making field, it follows that even when the participants in the decision-making process are in conflict about a wide range of issues, the one thing that unites them is their sex. Thus, even if there are areas of conflict between the actors, they all have a 'vested interest' in the maintenance of the patriarchal status quo. This is not necessarily to say that there is a plot on the part of the male-dominated establishment to reproduce and sustain a male supremacist structure and ideology. Nonetheless, in practice the maintenance of this structure and its associated ideology are be the consequences of their actions.

3 What is patriarchy?

Since we have claimed that we need to introduce the concept of patriarchy into any satisfactory explanatory model, the first task is to explain what this concept means. Broadly speaking, the term refers to a form of political power. But beyond this very general characterisa-tion, there is little agreement between feminist political theorists on the best way to understand the term. Debates between feminists revolve around such issues as whether in our society, the term should be used in its literal meaning of rule by the fathers; whether patriarchy is a universal feature of human society or is historically and culturally variable; whether patriarchal relations are found primarily in the family or whether social life as a whole is structured by patriarchal power; and what relationship exists between patriarchy or sexual domination on the one hand, and capitalism or class domination on the other. On none of these issues is there any consensus among contemporary feminists; and some have even claimed that problems with the concept are so great that it should be abandoned altogether. But others have argued that to follow such a course would mean that feminist political theory was deprived of the only concept at its disposal which refers specifically to the subjection of women, and which singles out that form of political right that all men exercise by virtue of being men. We *do* need a name for that particular power relationship, a name which singles out that relationship from other power relationships. If the concept of patriarchy is abandoned, then this power relationship has no name at all, and the study and awareness of patriarchy could all too easily slide back into obscurity beneath the conventional categories of political analyses.

How, then, should we understand the concept of patriarchy? Rather than discussing the *institution* of patriarchy, we will approach the topic by focusing on the slightly narrower idea of patriarchal *beliefs*. Here, a number of different ideas could be emphasised. One conception of patriarchal beliefs would focus entirely on their *content*. A belief would thus count as patriarchal if it portrayed women as inferior in some respect or other. A different strand in the idea of patriarchy would focus not on the content of the belief but on its *effects*. A belief would then count as patriarchal if the effects of the belief were systematically disadvantageous to women — and correlatively advantageous to men. A third strand would shift our attention from the content and the effects of the beliefs to its *origin*. If the belief is held (e.g. by men) *because* it has the effects which it does, *because* it brings advantages to men and disadvantages to women, it would count as patriarchal.

The concept of patriarchal belief which we will deploy utilises several of the above ideas. It defines patriarchal beliefs in terms of four features:

a such beliefs embody a stereotype of women
b the stereotype they embody is a negative one
c the stereotype was created by men
d the stereotype operates to women's disadvantage.

Since our strategy is to show that reference must be made to patriarchal beliefs and their influence if we are satisfactorily to explain the actions of policy-makers, we need to show that it is antecedently plausible to suppose that they hold such beliefs. we will do this by demonstrating how these beliefs are clearly evident in the elite discourses of the culture. The point here is that political elites are situated within a patriarchal society, and hence willy-nilly absorb society's values and beliefs. The next section will therefore look at some elite discourses, and show how they are riddled with patriarchal beliefs.

4 Patriarchal beliefs in elite discourses

In her book *The Creation of Feminist Consciousness*, Lerner, remarks:

> Briefly summarised the major assumptions about gender in patriarchal society are these: Men and women are essentially different creatures, not only in their biological equipment, but in their needs, capacities and functions. Men and women also differ in the way they were created and in the social function assigned to them by God. Men are 'naturally' superior, stronger and more rational, and are therefore designed to be dominant. From this it follows that men are political citizens and responsible for and representing the polity. Women are 'naturally' weaker, inferior in intellect and rational capacities, unstable emotionally and therefore incapable of political participation. They stand outside the polity . . . Men mediate between humans and God. Women reach God through the mediation of men. These unproven, unprovable assumptions are not, of course, laws of either nature or society, although they have often been so regarded and have even been incorporated into human law. They are operative at different levels, in different forms and with different intensity during various periods of history. Changes in the way in which these patriarchal assumptions are acted upon describe in fact changes in the status and position of women in a given period in a given society' (Lerner, 1993, p. 4).

The tracing of these kinds of beliefs and assumptions has been an important string to the bow of feminist political theorists. It is important because these beliefs and assumptions are used to define and construct civil society, and in so doing give authority and institutional power to the male rather than the female. Lerner (1993) points out that as far back as the philosophical writings of Aristotle it was clear that women were not considered to be capable of being political beings in the way that males were, and she further claims that 'Aristotle's misogynist assumptions remained virtually unchallenged and endlessly repeated for nearly two thousand years' (Lerner, 1993, p. 7). She claims that the same misogynistic beliefs can even be observed in the writings of the founding fathers of the American republic. What is important about these observations from the point of view of this thesis is that they demonstrate that firstly the beliefs and assumptions associated with patriarchy are well entrenched in the elite discourses of Western culture, and secondly, that the beliefs and assumptions have practical consequences in terms of the distribution of institutional power between the sexes, and the construction of political and civil order.

Many recent studies have demonstrated the prevalence of patriarchal beliefs in Western culture, and it is neither possible nor necessary within the confines of the present study to review all of this material. But some consideration *is* necessary in order to demonstrate that these beliefs are indeed endemic within Western culture, and that furthermore they are part of the academic, political and religious culture. This implies that the ideas are widely held as being 'valid' and 'natural'. We will therefore select as typical examples the two areas of religion and political theory.

One of the most powerful and influential sources of patriarchal beliefs is to be found within various world religions. Within Christianity in particular, one dominant model of women has been based on Eve. Eve is seen as the embodiment of human moral weakness, unable to abide by simple rules constructed by a good (male) God for human welfare, unable to resist the temptations of physical pleasure, and hence ultimately responsible for the 'fall of man'. This view of women as being both intellectually and morally weak has a clear history, traceable through European scholarly literature from at least as the Middle Ages onwards. Women as well as men have internalised these stereotypical beliefs about women and the 'nature' of women. One recent sign of these internalised beliefs, for example, is the recent controversy over the ordination of women. (For further details about patriarchal content of much religious ideology, see Mary Daly (1986)).

But religion is not the only place where examples of patriarchal beliefs can be found. If we turn to the writings of the most influential political theorists in the Western tradition, we will find a similar set of patriarchal assumptions. In the writings of Rousseau and Kant, the supposed weakness and political 'disorderliness' of women is invoked in order to exclude them from taking part in political activity. They are pronounced lacking in those capacities required for an individual to become a citizen. Contract theorists such as Locke and Rousseau seek to justify this conclusion by appeal to women's biological role in the family (coupled with moral and intellectual weakness). Men can be trusted to undertake the running of civil society because they possess 'reason' while women do not. (For further details, see Pateman (1989)).

It is clear that in both of these areas a stereotype of women has been created; that the stereotype is indeed negative; and that it has been created and perpetuated largely by men, even though it has also been internalised by women. So three of the four essential features of patriarchal beliefs are obviously present. What about the fourth condition, that the system of beliefs operate to women's disadvantage? That, too, can be shown, though we will wait until section 6 and the discussion of patriarchal power before we mention the relevant evidence.

What is revealed by the critical analysis provided by Daley, Pateman and others, is the extent to which past elite discourse about the nature of women operates on patriarchal assumptions we have referred to above. One of the main strands is that women are incapable of reason and abstract thinking, whereas men do possess these qualities. Since these are exactly the qualities individuals need if they are to take part in public life, it follows that it is men and not women who should dispose of public power.

It is also important to note the higher status accorded to rational thought over both 'non-rational' thought and physical labour of any sort. Jagger (1983) calls this division of the mental and the physical 'normative dualism'. She comments that of course both men and women have physical bodies and minds, but throughout western philosophical traditions women have consistently been portrayed as connected with or entangled with their bodies in a far more intimate way than has been the case with portrayals of men. Women's bodies are thought to commit them irrevocably to the biological reproduction of the species. Women are seen as being closer to nature. Men, by contrast are thought to express their creativity through the creation of culture. In short, then, the view expressed through normative dualism is that women are associated with nature and males with culture; women with the body and males with the mind.

In fact, however, this connection between female biological functions and body, and male biological characteristics and mind, is an arbitrary construction of patriarchy. Steinem (1984) considers how menstruation might be given entirely different connotations under patriarchy if it were the men who had to 'do' it; the entanglement with biology would be given higher status. If it were men and not women who menstruated, menstruation might be seen as a sign of male superiority, a monthly purification which meant that men alone could enter the priesthood. It would perhaps be seen as a biological link to the cycles of the moon and planets, a link which meant that men alone could be mathematicians or understand the patterns of the universe, a symbolic blood-letting that made men alone fit to be warriors and rulers.

What the above shows us is that, historically, patriarchal beliefs have been entrenched in at least two major strands (religion and politics) of the cultural traditions of western thought. It would therefore not be surprising if these values and beliefs were to be absorbed not only by those who dispose of public power, but also by those who engage in academic study of the beliefs. And when we turn to consider influential figures in our own century, we find confirmation of this hypothesis.

Freud, for example, considered women to be deprived by nature of the capacity for a clear-cut resolution of the Oedipal conflict. From this, he argued that women's super-ego — the heir to the Oedipus complex — was compromised: 'for women the level of what is ethically normal is different from what it is in men'(Freud, 1925, p. 259) Freud concluded that 'women show less sense of justice than men, they are less ready to submit to the exigencies of life, they are more often influenced by feelings or affection or hostility' [Frued, 1925, p. 260). Freud alleged that women's sense of justice is compromised because they seem simply to refuse to make moral judgements based on 'blind impartiality'.

The same assumptions reappear in the work of Piaget. In his account of the development of moral reasoning, girls appear to be not much more than a branch line, while boys provide the blueprint for the 'proper' development of moral reasoning (Piaget, 1932).

But perhaps the most striking modern example in elite 'academic' discourse of these entrenched patriarchal assumptions is to be found in the work of Kohlberg on moral development. Kohlberg's theory (1958, 1981) of six stages of moral development, which describe the processes through which individuals develop the ability to engage in moral reasoning from child to adult, is based on a study of 84 boys whose development Kohlberg closely traced for more than twenty years. Among those who failed to reach the highest stage of Kohlberg's scale of moral development are women, who seem unable to get past stage three.

The explanation of this 'inability' lies in the way Kohlberg ranked the various abilities which he was considering. Abstract reasoning comes at the top of the scale while helping and caring for others is often low down. (Gilligan points out that this is a very male way of ranking these abilities). In her study, which parallels Kohlberg's, Gilligan (1982), found that when children were given the same moral dilemmas as those in Kohlberg's study, the ways in which girls solved the problem were certainly different from the ways followed by boys. Boys tended to treat the dilemmas almost as a kind of mathematical (abstract) problem, whereas the girls 'instead saw a world comprised of relationships rather than of people standing alone, a world that coheres through human connection rather than through a system of rules' (p29). In other words, the way in which the girls dealt with the dilemma was as sophisticated as that used by the boys. But because being helpful and caring for others is ranked low on Kohlberg's scale, the girls' insistence on seeing the world in terms of relationships meant that Kohlberg's male-stream psychology judged the female variety of moral reasoning to be deficient. Gilligan concludes that men and women speak in 'different voices', and that because it is the males who set the agenda and make the rules, 'feminine logic' and reasoning is always going to be ignored. Men and women do not speak the same 'language', and they often engage in what Sabatier terms a 'dialogue of the deaf'. Gilligan comments:

> My research suggests that men and women may speak different languages that they assume are the same, using similar words to encode disparate experiences of self and social relationships. Because these languages share an overlapping moral vocabulary, they contain the propensity for systematic mistranslation . . . As we have listened to the voices of men and the theories of development that their experience informs, so have we come more recently to notice not only the silence of women but the difficulty in hearing what they say when they do speak' (Gilligan, 1982, p. 173).

What, then is the significance of these observations about women's ability to engage in abstract reasoning? What they show is that it is men who define what counts as 'proper' reasoning and 'proper' justice, and that consequently other kinds of reasoning, and other moral conceptions are regarded as deficient or even ignored altogether. It also suggests that the moral concepts which are underlie decision-making process are gendered. But the examination of the work of writers such as Pateman, Gilligan and Walby goes further than a simple demonstration that patriarchal attitudes and beliefs exist in the elite discourse of western culture. Pateman and Gilligan have both approached the analysis of the content of elite discourses by examining closely the underlying assumptions expressed through the texts of the various 'authorities' that they have chosen. The choice is not a random or accidental one. The writers (such as Freud, Kant, Hobbes etc) are pivotal in the development of 'western thought'. That is to say that Aristotles' theories of democracy and Freuds' theories about the nature of human beings, is not limited in its influence to the realms of psychology or democratic theory alone. The concepts, attitudes and values expressed in them 'seep out' into the wider field of academic and political activity. In order to make full use of their work, the method of textual analysis could be applied to the principal document concerned with this case study, ie the Forrest Report. For if they are correct then it should be possible to find some expression of patriarchal attitudes and beliefs within that text. As we shall see in chapter five, this is indeed the case. Walby's work, on the other hand, concentrates less on a textual analysis, and takes a more pragmatic view of the process of decision making. She points out that patriarchal attitudes can be clearly detected by the *consequences* that public policies have on the lives of women. The crucial point being that if a persistent bias can be observed in the outcomes of public policies, then this is not likely to be purely coincidence. *If* we live in a society where 'patriarchy rules', then we would expect to observe a distribution pattern of welfare (in its broadest sense) where overall, men benefit and women loose. She therefore asks this question with particular reference to those recent policy changes that have supposedly been implemented on womens' behalf. A discussion of the results has already taken place within these pages. By the same token, we shall ask, can the breast cancer screening programme be analysed in the same way? After all, it was a policy option which was 'marketed' as being in the interests of women. If this were true, then we would expect to observe some kind of benefit for the target population of women. But, as we shall see in chapter five, this was not the case.

Given the above evidence of the still-pervasive influence of patriarchal conceptions, we would naturally expect to find these conceptions informing the activities of many modern decision-making bodies. In particular, it would be a reasonable *initial* assumption to make when we look at the workings of the Forrest Committee to suppose that committee was not immune from the patriarchy which is endemic in the society from which the committee members were drawn. Whether this initial assumption is in fact confirmed would of course depend upon how the Forrest Committee actually behaved; and in the next chapter we will show this initial assumption receives ample empirical justification.

However, before we turn to that task, there is the second element which we mentioned to be considered, namely power. For it would be a mistake to think that patriarchal beliefs carry no implications about the distribution of power. It might be possible in theory for a group of people to hold patriarchal beliefs in a situation in which women were a dominant group (rather as it would be *possible* for anti-black beliefs to be held in a society in which blacks were in fact dominant). But in practice, patriarchal beliefs are almost invariably associated with positions of unequal power. They are found in situations in which men are dominant and women are subservient. Nor is this a coincidental correlation. Patriarchal beliefs are *naturally expressed in* power relationships, and they serve to legitimate both the general existence of an unequal distribution of power, and also more particularly the detailed ways in which that power is exercised. Putting the matter over-simply: women are declared *properly* subservient to men; and men then use their dominance to act against the interests of women. It is at this point that the fourth condition in our explanation of what patriarchal beliefs are becomes important. In order to complete our understanding of patriarchal beliefs, we therefore need to say something about the best way to understand these power relationships.

5 Power

Power comes in a variety of forms. These forms can vary in their effectiveness, and also in the degree to which they are observable. Among the forms of power which Wrong, for example, distinguishes are force, manipulation, persuasion, and authority (which in turn comes in a number of varieties) (Wrong 1979). Although we might initially think that force is the paradigm form of power, it is in fact the *least* effective form of power over a long period of time. In order to legitimate their position, 'power holders' ideally need the co-operation and consent of the oppressed; and therefore notions of authority, persuasion and manipulation come to the fore. This is a point that has been emphasised by writers as diverse as Wrong (1979), Arendt (1992) and Pateman (1989). Arendt, for example, suggests that power is something that is the property not so much of an individual, but rather of a group which 'acts in concert'. She therefore sees the basis of power to lie in a contract between free and equal parties by means of which they place themselves under mutual obligation (Arendt, 1992).

The idea that power can be exercised in these non-violent ways goes back to the Marxian idea of ideology as a form of social control. In our day, this conception of the exercise of power has been developed by theorists such as Althusser who urged that no class can hold power for any length of time simply by the use of force. Ideological control provides a far more effective means of maintaining class rule. If members of the subject class accept their position as normal and legitimate, they will be unlikely seriously to challenge the ruling class dominance — the subject class 'contracts in', as Pateman (1988) puts it in the feminist case. Maintenance of class rule, according to Marxists, is best achieved through ideological control. More specifically, the instruments of this ideological control are the 'Ideological State Apparatuses', which include the mass media, the law, religion, and education. Each of these instills the values and beliefs of the dominant ideology into the subject class. This then enables the ruling class to exercise power in their own interest without any reliance on force. Their ideological domination ensures the complicity and acquiescence of subservient classes, precisely by hiding from those classes the real nature of the power that is being exercised over them.

In a parallel way, we will claim, patriarchal beliefs, which are also maintained by institutions in society (such those as mentioned earlier) function as dominant ideologies and are a means by which men exercise power over women. They secure the complicity and acquiescence of women by making women think that their inferior position is 'natural'. It is natural because it is God-ordained; or derives from *intrinsic* differences between men and women (for example in terms of rationality, morality, etc) (see section 4 above). Because the inferiority is seen as being thus intrinsic to the very idea of different sexes, it is possible to portray attempts to change it as at best a waste of effort, and at worst socially and individually disastrous, raising expectations that cannot possibly be met.

In the next section, we will trace out in more detail how patriarchal power in particular is manifested.

6 Patriarchy and power

One writer who is broadly sympathetic to the ideas sketched above, and who has focused on patriarchal power in particular, is Sylvia Walby. She argues that patriarchal power is exercised through a number of interlocking channels (Walby, 1990, p. 20). Consequently, she claims, the term 'power' needs to be conceptualised at different levels of abstraction; and she therefore distinguishes six areas of patriarchal power:

a the patriarchal means of production
b patriarchal relations in the workplace
c patriarchal relations in the state
d male violence
e patriarchal relations in sexuality
f patriarchal relations in cultural institutions.

Clearly some of these categories relate to those suggested by Althusser. For example, Walby's 'cultural institutions' are analogous to Althussers' mass media, religion and education; and patriarchal relations in the state correspond to Althussers' category of the law. Where Walby's typology departs from an Althusserian or Marxist analysis of class domination is in its inclusion of the personal aspects of women's lives, for example sexuality; and this moves the concept away from a purely public conception of power, towards a more private one, or at least one with private dimensions. In other words, unlike class domination, patriarchal power exists, and is practised, in the private sphere of the family, with men exercising power over their wives and children. And her reference to male violence re-introduces the idea of power as force that we noticed earlier. But, important though these 'private' exercises of power are for a full understanding of patriarchy, we will leave them on one side here, as my focus is on the exercise of patriarchal power within the public arena. In what follows, we will first outline the way in which the state exercises patriarchal power, and then in the next section, we will focus more specially on the patriarchy within the medical profession.

7 Patriarchal power and the state

The important fact for our present purposes is that the state is overwhelmingly male-dominated, or to be more accurate is dominated by white, middle-class, middle-aged men (Burstyn, 1983). Whether this means that policies are patriarchal is a question that feminists have answered with a resounding 'yes'. As Walby notes:

The state is patriarchal as well as being capitalist and racist. While being a site for struggle and not a monolithic entity, the state has a systematic bias towards patriarchal interests in its policies and actions . . . The state is systematically structured in a way that makes it appropriate to regard it as patriarchal. Its actions are more often in men's interests than women's (Walby, 1990, p. 21).

Walby concerns herself primarily with policy outputs rather than with an examination of the decision-making process. But after a careful examination of a number of areas of policy-making, she concludes that all the major changes in the areas of divorce, employment, welfare provision, culture, sexuality, and violence have served the interests of men rather than women. This has been the case, even in respect of changes which at first sight are to the advantage of women. For example, a number of changes have tended to reduce the extent to which women are confined to the private sphere, and have encouraged them into the public sphere of employment; and equal opportunity legislation has been passed to ensure that women do not suffer unfair sexual discrimination. These changes might at first seem to go against the idea that the state's activities are comprehensively patriarchal. But in fact this series of changes has not brought about any major improvement in the position of women. The equal opportunity legislation, for example, is widely considered to have had only a marginal impact. Coupled with this, women as single parents find themselves in an economically perilous position, with low levels of state provision, both in terms of state benefits and also in terms of childcare provision, or tax relief on child-care fees. Furthermore, changes in legislation governing part-time employment have meant that in those areas of the job market where women tend to be employed (i.e. part-time, unskilled, and semi-skilled occupations), work has become notoriously insecure, badly paid, and non-unionised.

Thus it would be a mistake to take at face value those recent changes in state policy which are apparently in women's interests. Such changes, while appearing to be more attentive to the needs and rights of women, in fact simply mask a deeper tendency to reinforce patriarchal power.

This view of the state as an instrument of patriarchal power is also shared by liberal feminists such as Eisenstein (1981). She reiterates the point made above about the parallels between a feminist and a Marxist critique of the state, and goes on to argue that it is men's economic power which gives them control of the state and allows them to perpetuate the subordination of women. Thus, the election of one or two token women into positions of government responsibility does not significantly change the power position, so long as men retain economic power. According to this view, the state is an instrument of patriarchy which cannot be trusted to enforce women's rights, and women owe no allegiance to it.

Eisenstein suggests that the practice of contemporary liberal feminists will force them eventually to develop a feminist theory of the state. This theory will have to recognise that the state is not a neutral arbiter between conflicting social groups but rather is 'the condensation of a balance of forces', (Eisenstein, 1981) a balance in which one of the strongest forces is male dominance. Eisenstein states that this realisation will be forced upon liberal feminists; for as they continue to struggle for state-instituted reforms, they will discover that the 'motive of the state via liberal feminism is to keep women in their place as secondary wage earners and as mothers' (Eisenstein, 1981, p. 226).

What both Eisenstein and Walby are saying is that patriarchal power exists in a variety of forms. Walby draws attention to a theoretical distinction between 'public' and 'private' patriarchy, while Eisenstein's focus is more upon the state as a kind of instrument of patriarchal power which stands more or less as a 'thing' in itself. Both authors make implicit reference to the existence within this patriarchal power structure of a system of beliefs that conforms to our earlier conceptualisation of what a patriarchal belief consists of.

This view of the state as an instrument of patriarchal power is one that has been well-documented by many other contemporary feminists; and feminist critiques of social policy in particular have produced a wealth of evidence which supports the notion that women are ill-served in a variety of areas of public policy. This is the theme pursued by, for example, the contributors to Hearn et al. (1989, p. 179) who conclude that:

> We have come to see both the regularity of patterns of [male] domination in organisations and the ever increasing subtlety of the processes whereby organisations are sexualized . . . . The subtlety of these processes in no way dilutes the patterns of domination . . . on the contrary it is difficult to over-estimate the depth and complexity of the ways in which dominant forms are produced and reproduced, not just in the broad structuring of organisations but also in the minutiae of organisations (p. 179).

For other writers who endorse and document the patriarchal

nature of state activity include Zaretsky (1976); Wilson (1977); Cockburn (1979); Doyal (1979); Austerberry (1981); Flax (1983); Smart (1984); Pascall (1986).

What is not being claimed here is that all individuals (or groups) always and in every case act in accordance with their beliefs. There are many reasons why this mismatch between belief and action may happen, but when we examine decision-making of the kind we are here concerned with, it seems reasonable to suppose that a consistent and regular bias in favour of one group at the expense of another, over a long period of time, represents the reflection of what Sabatier calls deep core beliefs, and that these can be reliably invoked as a 'cause' of policy preferences even if the beliefs concerned (in this case patriarchal beliefs) are not explicitly expressed by the actors involved.

When we refer to the use of patriarchal power in this context, we are clearly not talking about what Wrong calls 'force'. We mentioned earlier the way in which there is a consensus among writers with very different perspectives that force is an inefficient means of control, and how Arendt in particular had sought to replace this with the idea of contract. Pateman extends this idea of contract to cover the case of women in particular. She argues that women 'contract in' to the exercise of patriarchal power. But, Pateman insists, this is not a true contract, because women are neither free nor equal parties to the contract. The contract is drawn up by men, and its terms favour their interests:

> In the natural condition 'all men are born free' and are equal to each other, they are 'individuals'. This presupposition of contract doctrine generates a profound problem: how in such a condition can the government of one man by another ever be legitimate? how can political right exist? The relationship must arise through agreement . . . contract is seen as the paradigm of free agreement. But women are not born free, women have no natural freedom . . . . with the exception of Hobbes, the classic theorists claim that women naturally lack the attributes and capacities of 'individuals'. Sexual difference is political difference, sexual difference is the difference between freedom and subjection (Pateman, 1988, p. 6).

One of the questions which this analysis raises is why women would 'contract in' to a system that patently operates against their interests? A possible answer is that women have a 'false perception' of what is really in their interests. This leads us into the tricky area of

103

what 'interests' really are, and how we know what is in our interests. Lukes (1986, p. 5), following Joel Feinberg, suggests that we can define interests as:

> A miscellaneous collection consisting of all those things in which one has a stake, whereas one's interest in the singular, one's personal interest consists in the harmonious advancement of all one's interests in the plural (Lukes, 1986, p. 5).

Having defined interests, Lukes next divides them into two broad categories: first, interests in an individual's ultimate goals and aspirations; and secondly, interests in the necessary means to those ultimate goals. Lukes then poses the question of how interests so defined relate to beliefs. He concludes that:

> The answer is complex, but there are a few points worth stressing. First it seems on the face of it, odd for someone to believe that he or she has an interest in something but not want it. On the other hand, secondly, one can fail to want something that is in one's interests either because one does not know that it is in one's interests, or because one does not know that it is causally related to what is in one's interests (Lukes, 1986, p. 6).

What this discussion reveals is the close connection between wants, desires, beliefs and interests. But clearly a perception of what is in one's interests can be traced back in some way or another to one's beliefs. As mentioned before, this is the point at which for Althusser and for many feminist writers, the role of discourses and ideology becomes crucial. For Althusser, the ideological state apparatuses create false class consciousness because the oppressed class internalises the values and beliefs of the capitalist ruling class. Many feminist writers believe that in a parallel way, this is exactly the role played by patriarchal ideology. Dominant discourses promulgate patriarchal values and beliefs and both men and women are persuaded by them: they are internalised by the oppressed class (to borrow a term from marxism), and this plays a key role in the production and reproduction of patriarchal power.

Of course, it could be argued that false consciousness is not a useful concept for explaining people's behaviour: it implies that the observer knows better than the subject what is in their interests. The difficulties of invoking a notion of false class consciousness to explain 'contracting in' is one that has been discussed at length by both feminists and other political theorists at some length (see e.g. Herzog (1956); Radcliffe-Richards (1982)).

Having now outlined in general terms the way in which patriarchal beliefs express themselves in power relationships within the public arena as a whole, we now want to look at the same issue in relation to the medical profession in particular.

8 Patriarchy, power, and the medical profession

There are a number of characteristics of the medical profession which might plausibly be seen as the expression of patriarchal attitudes (for example, the difficulties of women seeking promotion to senior levels). But here we want to focus on the doctor/patient relationship in particular as one involving the exercise of patriarchal power.

A male doctor's relation to his patients in fact embodies several power relationships other than those which derive from patriarchy, and these now need to be disentangled.

In the first place, simply in virtue of their roles, the patient needs the doctor more than the doctor needs the patient. Although the doctor of course needs some patients or other, he does not need any particular patient. It is the patient who comes to him in the role of supplicant, not the doctor who supplicates the patient. This immediately gives the doctor a power over the patient. (This is not to deny that the power may be exercised benignly.)

In the second place, the doctor is the 'expert' and the patient is 'the ignorant one'. This notion of expertise here has several strands. The doctor can diagnose the ailment, can offer a prognosis, can recommend treatment, none of which is possible for the patient. Furthermore, in doing this, the doctor resorts to a language which is the language of an elite, and incomprehensible to the patient, unless the doctor provides a translation. This knowledge dimension is another respect in which the doctor holds power over the patient.

Thirdly, and following on from the first two points, the doctor is 'active', and patient 'passive' (the latter being an etymological tautology!). The patient presents himself/herself as a physical body to be 'managed' by the doctor. It is the doctor who renders the patient unconscious, controls blood pressure, oxygen levels, etc. and who cuts, drills, sews, etc. the patient's body, while the patient merely endures whatever treatment the doctor decides to administer.

Fourthly, the different roles are backed up by legal sanctions. It is given to the doctor alone to authorise most forms of treatment, whether this consists of signing a prescription form, declaring the patient fit for work, referring him/her to a consultant at a hospital, or treating the patient's body in ways which would be regarded as criminal assault if produced by anyone else. It is a criminal offence to 'impersonate a doctor', or for a 'lay' person to carry out 'medical' procedures. For example, a woman's partner may not deliver a baby 'on purpose', and indeed there have been prosecutions for doing so, when the women involved refused point blank to go into hospital.

The point of distinguishing these aspects of the power relationship between doctors and patients is that these four aspects are present whether the patient is a man or woman. Hence they need to be distinguished from the specifically *patriarchal* forms of power which doctors possess. What we need to focus on therefore, are forms of power relationship which are *peculiar* to female patients.

One natural area to look would therefore be in relation to types of treatment offered only to women. The whole area of obstetrics and gynaecology, for example, is of particular interest because clearly it is an area of 'medical science' which is practised exclusively upon female patients, by an almost exclusively male profession. Savage (1986) supplies some striking statistics illustrating this imbalance:

> Of the 764 consultant obstetricians and gynaecologists in England and Wales, there are 88 women, (11.5%). This is reflected within the committee structure of the RCOG where 10% of the members are women. However, in 1986 only one woman was elected to the council, and all but one of the 26 committees are chaired by men . . . The incongruity of a speciality devoted to women being almost totally controlled by men has always struck me forcefully (Savage, 1986, p. 59).

Let us consider, then, hysterectomy as an example. This has become one of the most frequently performed operations. It has been estimated that in England and Wales, by the age of 75 one in five women has had a hysterectomy (Cape, 1981). And yet these major operations often have only dubious value in medical terms. In her study of hysterectomy, Cape comments:

> Sometimes it's used as a form of sterilisation. It's also advocated for what the medical profession term 'neurosis'. One woman told us that her doctor advised a hysterectomy partly because her womb was prolapsed, but also because he thought it might 'cure' her 'nervous problems' and stop her being so 'obsessed' with her

'ailments'. Dr James Simmonds, executive vice president of the American Medical Association, told a congressional hearing in 1977 that anxiety relief justifies a hysterectomy for a woman with an extreme fear of cervical cancer (Cape, 1981, p. 38).

Some feminist writers (e.g. Daly (1984)) see this burgeoning of hysterectomies (and other major operations on women) as a kind of symbolic mutilation of the female body — a kind of castration; and Deborah Larner has pointed out that for several years gynaecologists have been promoting hysterectomies as a 'simple solution for everything from backaches to contraception'.

A parallel development can be seen in the increase in the number of births occurring through caesarian section. The number has more than tripled since 1970. Research suggests that the reason for this increase does not lie with concern for the safety of the mother or her baby, but rather with the convenience of the obstetrician, and the higher status associated with the surgical delivery of a baby compared with the 'natural' delivery (Oakley (1986)). Even with a vaginal delivery, women are often forced to lie in a supine 'stranded beetle' position which is difficult and uncomfortable for the woman, but convenient for the obstetrician. Furthermore, the use of complicated technological equipment makes it impossible for women to control the process through which they give birth.

Another area of medical practice which affects exclusively women is breast cancer screening, where a similar bias can be observed. Here too we find that an almost exclusively male team of 'experts' is concerned with the screening of a (healthy) patient population which is exclusively female. Skrabanek comments on the eagerness of the male experts to engage in breast cancer screening in the following terms:

> There is something rather strange or funny about this pressure to implement breast cancer screening coming from all these late middle aged men. Actually there is something peculiar that as far as screening is concerned it's actually limited to the screening of the sexual organs of women, usually younger women. If there were a similar suggestion that for cancers in men that were as common as breast cancer in older women — testicular cancer for example — a similar proposition would not go down very well with either the male population or be considered as a serious option by the medical profession. If you were to tell men that this was a preventable disease by screening, but maybe you have to

do ten unnecessary testicular biopsies or maybe to do some unnecessary orchidectomies — men would say you must be joking (personal interview, 1993)

In the light of facts such as those outlined above, some radical feminists have concluded that the primary object of patriarchal power is the control of women's bodies (see Firestone (1971) and Brownmiller (1975); and medical practice offers the perfect medium through which this control can be exercised, and given a 'scientific' authority and status. March echoes this idea when she writes that:

Feminist materialists are more likely to turn to religions and *medical institutions* as the primary agencies solidifying, enforcing and reproducing male control and misogyny (March, 1979 p. 269, italics added).

Daly also agrees with the line taken by Brownmiller and Firestone, but goes further and concludes that the American profession is not only misogynistic but also sadistic:

It's obvious that there is a breast surgery craze, and that this is connected with the breast fetishism of the entire culture. Sadistic surgery is targeted at that which symbolises the female to the fetishist. It keeps women pure, that is terrified, victimised, docile (Daly, 1979, p. 244).

Whether Daly is right about the medical profession being both misogynistic and sadistic is open to debate. But what is clear, and is very widely accepted by contemporary feminist writers, are the spread and depth of patriarchal actions and attitudes throughout the medical profession. Further, these actions and attitudes are the expression of (and also gives rise to) patriarchal *policies*.

What conclusions, then, can we draw from the discussion so far, about the role of patriarchal beliefs and power in the policy-making process? Two main points in particular need to be emphasised:

A. Because policy makers are situated within a patriarchal society, they acquire the patriarchal beliefs which we have found are widespread in elite discourses. This is not to imply a conscious conspiracy on the part of policy-makers as a whole to act in a male supremacist way (although a few may be consciously conspiratorial). The point is rather that the policy outcomes are an expression of a comprehensive male bias, which stems from a set of largely unconscious patriarchal preferences which are endemic to the world of policy-making.

B. These patriarchal beliefs are expressed in a series of power relationships. Typically in the public arena, this power is not exercised through force, but by obtaining the complicity in women in their subservient role.

It follows from this that any satisfactory model of decision-making, particularly in domains in which women's interests are at stake, must take into account the role played by both patriarchal beliefs and power relationships. Armed with these conclusions, we can now turn again to the Sabatier model, and suggest some necessary changes.

9 Sabatier revisited

The main changes required concern two main areas: the prevalence of patriarchal beliefs; and the distribution of power which follows on from those beliefs. But we will start with two modifications which are more a matter conceptual tidying up than of substance.

First, Sabatier's threefold division of beliefs into deep core, near core and secondary aspects is unnecessary and is arbitrary. A better conceptualisation would see all beliefs ranged on a spectrum of entrenchment, or degree of resistance to change. Those which Sabatier calls deep core will be very highly entrenched; the near core will be fairly well-entrenched; and the secondary will be relatively weakly entrenched. But there is only a *difference of degree* (of entrenchment) between the deep core and the secondary. To suppose that there are three (and only three) levels of resistance to change is psychologically implausible and theoretically unwarranted. But for the sake of convenience in what follows, we will continue to speak of 'deep core' etc beliefs, but this phrase needs to be understood in the way we have just indicated.

Furthermore, there is no reason to assume that all and only the deep core beliefs will concern deeply felt matters of moral principle. The most highly entrenched beliefs *can* include matters of moral principle, but can also include a wide variety of other kinds of cognitive commitment (for example scientific, religious, aesthetic, etc). However, we can agree with Sabatier that *within the area of policy conflict*, the relevant deep core beliefs are likely to concern matters that

109

are, in a wide sense of the term, moral.

Let us now turn to the more substantial modifications. Sabatier stresses the *variety* of deep core beliefs held by different groups; and this variety is important to his account for two reasons. First, it is partly because of their shared deep core beliefs that a number of individuals will belong to a single coalition; and hence it partly in terms of differing deep core beliefs that different coalitions are identified. Secondly, Sabatier tries to use this variety in deep core beliefs to explain the conflicts which emerge between the rival groups. The fact of variety among deep core beliefs thus has both an identificatory role (i.e. identifying the set of individuals belonging to a single coalition); and also an explanatory role (i.e. explaining the conflict between coalitions).

But we have now seen good reason to think that the picture is more complicated than Sabatier allows. As section 4 of this chapter showed, patriarchal beliefs are very widely disseminated in the culture, both in classic historical texts found in influential areas of life, such as politics and religion, and also in contemporary writings, including those by 'scientific' figures (such as Freud, Kohlberg, et al.). This means that it is antecedently highly probable (i.e. antecedently to seeing the policies supported by different advocacy coalitions) that *rival* coalitions may in fact *share* patriarchal assumptions. Of course, different coalitions will still hold other deep core beliefs in terms of which the coalitions can be distinguished from each other. But the fact that they may also share deep core patriarchal beliefs is important because it implies that *no matter which coalition turns out to be most influential*, the policy output from that area is likely to be at least tinged with patriarchy.

Secondly, let us consider a situation in which there are a number of rival coalitions. They will by definition be distinguished in terms of the differing deep core beliefs which they hold. But (as suggested above) we now have some reason to expect that one deep core belief which will be common to most if not all of the coalitions will be a belief in patriarchy. So far, it might seem simply that the coalitions share some of their core beliefs, and differ in others. But *given the content of patriarchal beliefs*, we can now see that from a woman's perspective it is very likely that the (patriarchal) beliefs which the coalitions all share are much more significant than the (non-patriarchal) beliefs about which they differ. In other words, what the coalitions have in common is more important than what differentiates them. This point can be neatly illustrated by focusing on the question of the access to the policy arena which the different policy groupings achieve.

110

Sabatier assumes that any group with an interest in an issue area can become involved in the policy subsystem, and thus affect its output, providing it has the resources (typically financial) and that it has some expertise in the area. It is true that he qualifies this claim in respect of the smaller coalitions. If they remain small, they have little chance of affecting policy on their own. They often therefore tend to become absorbed by the larger groups. Once an advocacy coalition becomes a 'member' of a policy subsystem, it can engage in the elite discourse and conflict. Further, it is also true that Sabatier does recognise that in some cases a very powerful advocacy coalition may dominate the elite discourse to such an extent that it can ensure that other groups are in practice excluded. For example, the RSPCA may dominate the policy subsystem concerned with animal rights, and although some other groups may be 'admitted' into the policy subsystem, other groups are not. The Animal Liberation Front, for example, is not regarded as being a 'respectable' organisation. Their beliefs concerning the 'rights' of animals may be very similar to the RSPCA, but because they are excluded from the 'official' policy subsystem, it is very difficult for them to engage in elite expert discourse on the matter.

So Sabatier does recognise that the policy arena is not always a level playing field where all groups, large and small, meet each other on equal terms. But he seems to think that the barriers to a group becoming part of the policy sub-system are of a practical kind, and do not have any ideological dimension.

But in the light of our discussion of patriarchy earlier in this chapter, we can now see the need to revise this picture. Firstly, we need to recognise that there is an ideological aspect to the question of who is admitted to the policy subsystem. There is an uncontroversial sense of this claim, a sense in which Sabatier can allow that it says something true. But there is also a sense which goes beyond what his model recognises. The uncontroversial sense is this: since he thinks that membership of advocacy coalitions is defined in terms of their shared deep core (ideological) beliefs, he can of course allow the relevance of an ideological dimension. It is relevant (in his eyes) in determining which coalition a contributor to a policy area will naturally ally with.

But there is a second and deeper way in which the ideological belief in patriarchy is relevant. Patriarchy (as we have seen in section 4 typically contains the belief that women are intellectually and morally inferior to men (men are creatures of reason, women of emotion, etc). This means that patriarchal core beliefs *implicitly exclude women from the policy arena altogether.* It is not so much that they are excluded from this or that particular coalition on the grounds that they do not share the requisite core beliefs. It is rather that patriarchy excludes them because it says that they suffer 'by nature' from incapacities which make them unfit to belong to *any* coalition which is going to be active in the policy arena.

Further, if certain groups can be excluded physically from the policy subsystem, they can also be excluded from the process of policy oriented learning. The important issue here is that certain kinds of information do not have the necessary credibility, and may be either ignored completely or denounced as inferior or mistaken. This may completely change the nature of the 'learning' or 'knowledge' that emerges from the policy subsystem, and since the policy subsystem is regarded as being the expert elite, the knowledge that they produce has the status of 'authority' while knowledge produced from other sources does not have this status, however carefully researched and prepared it may be.

This ability to exclude certain groups from the policy subsystem seriously undermines the validity of the policy oriented learning that the policy subsystem generates. It means that continuing debate within the policy arena is unlikely to produce any convergence on 'the truth', i.e. on polices which take account of all the relevant information. Rather, information and knowledge is *selected* by the policy sub-system, and it is selected because it meshes with the pre-existing deep core beliefs. This means that knowledge and information are used in a highly instrumental way by the whole policy subsystem in concert with each other. What conflict there is, tends to focus on what Sabatier would call secondary aspects and *not* over 'deep core' beliefs.

In the light of considerations like these, it would entirely reasonable to think that what *unites* a set of rival advocacy coalitions who share patriarchal beliefs will be much more significant for women than the various other core beliefs in terms of which the coalitions are distinguished one from another, and which are the focus of attention in a 'pure Sabatier' approach.

In summary then, the revised model of Sabatier appears thus:

1 The three fold division into deep core, is abandoned in favour of a continuum of degrees of entrenchment; and it is recognised that there is no correlation between the degree of entrenchment of some belief and its content. Deeply entrenched belief *can* be concerned with non-value matters.

2 Given the all-pervasive nature of patriarchal thinking in our society,

there is a standing assumption that one of the deep core beliefs held by all advocacy coalitions will be a belief in patriarchy. This assumption is of course defensible: it is certainly *possible* for a coalition to emerge which embraces non- or anti-patriarchal views. But that this possibility is realised would have to be demonstrated in each particular case.

3 Because the *content* of patriarchal beliefs declares women unfitted to participate in the arena of expert discourse and decision-taking, most coalitions are bound to seem from a woman's point of view to be in fundamental agreement with each other over what is perhaps the most important issue in any area of informed debate, namely who is to be admitted to the debate in the first place.

4 This exclusion of women from the arena of expert debate has two implications which are missing in the original Sabatier model. First, it means that a patriarchal screen filters out and discards pieces of relevant evidence, simply because they do not come from sources approved of within the patriarchal ideology. Secondly, and partly as a result of distortion in the inflow of information, there is also a deformation in the outcome: the policy-oriented learning which Sabatier presents as 'objective' learning is ideologically warped.

References

Arendt, H; (1970); *On Violence*, Brace and World, New York

Arendt, H; (1958); *The Human Condition*, University of Chicago Press, Chicago.

Austerberry, H., and Watson, S; (1981); 'A Womans Place: A Feminist Approach to Housing in Britain', *Feminist Review*, Summer Edition.

Brownmiller, S; (1977); *Against Our Will*, Penguin, Harmondsworth.

Burstyn, V; (1983); 'Masculine dominance and the State'. *Socialist Register*, pp. 45-89.

Cape, K; (1981); 'Wombloss', in *Womens Health A Spare Rib Reader*, Pandora Press, London.

Cockburn, C; (1977); *The Local State: The Management of Cities and People*, Pluto Press, London.

Daly, M; (1984); *Gyn/ecology: The Metaethics of Radical Feminism*, Womens' Press, London.

Daly, M; (1986); *Beyond God the Father*, Womens' Press, London.

Doyle, L., and Pennell, I; (1979); *The Political Economy of Health*, Pluto Press, London.

Eisenstein, Z; (1981); *The Radical Future of Liberal Feminism*, Longman, New York.

Feinberg, J; (1984); *Harm to Others*, Oxford University Press, New York.

Firestone, S; (1979); *The Diatectic of Sex*, Womens Press, London.

Flax, J; (1983); 'The Family in Contemporary Feminist Though, a Critical Review', in J. B. Elshtain (ed) *The Family in Political Thought*, Harvester, Brighton.

Gilligan, C; (1982); *In a Different Voice*, Harvard University Press, Cambridge, Mass.

Hearn, J., Sheppard, D., Tancred-Sherrif, P., and Burrell, G; (eds); (1989); *The Sexuality of Organisations*, Sage, London.

Herzog, D; (1989); *Happy Slaves: A Critique of Consent Theory*, University of Chicago Press, Chicago.

Jagger, A; (1983); *Feminist Politics and Human Nature*, Harvester Press, Brighton.

Kohlberg, L; (1981); *The Philosophy of Moral Development: Moral Stages and the Idea of Justice.* Harper and Row, London.

Lovenduski, J; (1989); *Mens Studies Modified*.

Oakley, A; (1986); *The Captured Womb*, Basil Blackwell, Cambridge.

Pascall, G; (1986); *Social Policy: A Feminist Analysis*, Tavistock, London.

Pateman, C; (1989); *The Disorder of Women: Democracy, Feminism and Political Theory*, Polity Press, Cambridge.

Pateman, C; (1988); *The Sexual Contract*, Polity Press, Cambridge.

Piaget, J; (1932); *The Moral Judgement of the Child*, Routledge and Keegan Paul, London.

Radcliffe-Richards, J; (1982); *The Sceptical Feminist*, Pluto Press, London.

Savage, W; (1986); *A Savage Enquiry*, Virago Press, London.

Smart, C; (1984); *The Ties That Bind: Law, Marriage and the Reproduction of Patriarchal Relations*, Routledge and Keegan Paul, London.

Steinem, G; (1984); *Outrageous Acts and Everyday Rebellions*, Fontana, London.

Walby, S; (1990); *Theorising Patriarchy*, Basil Blackwell, Oxford.

Wilson, E; (1977); *Women and the Welfare State.* Tavistock, London.

Wrong, D; (1979); *Power its Forms and Bases*, Basil Blackwell, Oxford.

Zaretsky, E; (1976); *Capitalism, The Family and Personal Life*, Pluto, London.

5 A feminist model applied

In the previous chapter, one of the principle concerns was to define what was meant by patriarchal beliefs, and to demonstrate that such beliefs are prevalent in the elite discourses of Western intellectual life. What was revealed was not only that the beliefs and attitudes associated with patriarchy are widespread, but also that these beliefs and attitudes typically are embedded in a set of power relationships. More specifically, it was shown that these patriarchal beliefs and power relationships are endemic in the medical profession. Since patriarchal beliefs are causally efficacious, it follows that reference needs to be made to them in the explanation of certain types of social phenomena. That both beliefs and power relationships must affect the decision making process seems obvious, what is a matter of debate is exactly how and in what ways this takes place. As was mentioned in Chapter Three, the use of models of decision making can cause some elements of the 'story' to be overlooked, while others are highlighted. In the previous chapter, we examined one element that had been consistently overlooked by the models of decision making so far deployed, ie the concept of patriarchy. The chapter concluded with a sketch in general terms of how these considerations about the nature and influence of patriarchal beliefs could be incorporated within a Sabatier-style explanation. The task of this chapter is to apply the general form of explanation which we have arrived at to the Forrest Committee in particular, and then to trace out the consequences for our understanding of the Report which the Committee produced.

In doing this, we will first show that the attribution of patriarchal beliefs to the Forrest Committee *in particular* is plausible. Secondly, we will outline what predictions one would derive from the revised Sabatier model which was propounded in chapter four. Thirdly, we will show how these predictions are confirmed by the actual behaviour of the committee, thus supporting the explanatory power of the model. And finally, we will also suggest briefly how the model could be extended to cover other areas of medical policy-making.

1 Patriarchy within the Forrest Committee

Having already noted the prevalence of patriarchal beliefs in elite life in general, and in the medical profession in particular, all that needs to be done here is to point to the wholly orthodox training and professional background of the members of the Committee. All of the principal members of the Forrest Committee had worked throughout their professional lives in institutions which are highly regarded within the medical profession. For example, Patrick Forrest himself had been Professor of Clinical Surgery at Edinburgh for several years before the creation of the Working Group and had established himself as a leading expert on breast cancer and breast cancer screening. Furthermore, he was a very active campaigner for breast cancer screening. At the time the working group was created, he had been a member of the Breast Cancer Research Sub-committee, the Scottish Advisory Committee on breast cancer screening and the Cancer Research Campaign. The other members of the Committee had similar backgrounds. All were trained at mainstream medical schools, all were respected staff members of established institutions, and all were also involved in a number of committees and groups concerned with breast cancer screening. None of them had any reputation for challenging patriarchal assumptions. Their background, in short, was exclusively of an entirely orthodox kind from within a solidly patriarchal profession. It is, then, a reasonable working hypothesis that deep and widespread assumptions found within the profession as a whole may have been at work in the Committee's thinking on the topic of breast cancer screening, and may have played a significant role in the Report which the Committee produced.

Further, it is reasonable to think that these patriarchal attitudes would have mutual encouragement within the environment of the Forrest Committee, for the members of the committee had all worked closely together before. Before Forrest, there had been four principal committees concerned with breast cancer, and the overlap between the membership of these committees is striking. Dr Joan Austoker, who ran the Oxford arm of the UK trial, noted the smallness of the breast cancer screening community:

> You go to all these various [breast cancer screening] committee meetings and steering groups, and they're all the same people, the same people keep turning up over and over again, and its been like that for years (personal interview, 1993).

The table (appendix 5) demonstrates the full extent of this overlap, and the 'incestuous' nature of the medical community concerned with screening.

It was not only in shared membership of a series of committees that this community would have become professionally intimate. They had also been working together for a number of years, in research and publication. Between 1970 and 1986 when the committee was set up, there were no fewer than sixteen joint research projects and articles (a full list of publications can be found in appendix 2. The importance of this system of interconnections must not be underrated. The significance is twofold. In the first place, it means that in the years prior to the creation of the Working Group, the members of this influential little 'community' of breast cancer experts had had plenty of time to hammer out a consensus position over the issues of the management and diagnosis of breast cancer and also the usefulness of a national breast cancer screening programme. Secondly, this shared history and shared knowledge of each other's views needs to be borne in mind in connection not just with the final recommendations of the committee, but also with the original selection of committee members. The committee's terms of reference required it to consider whether a breast screening programme was advisable, and Forrest as chair was given the authority to choose the other members of the committee. Given the prior relationship between the committee members which we have noted above, Forrest would have known before he made the selection what conclusions the committee members were likely to come to. The point here is not of course to suggest any sort of professional impropriety. It is rather to locate some *unconscious* but nevertheless important determinants both of the selection process, and ultimately of the committee's recommendations.

Another example of these important, but nonetheless unconscious, determinants is that the members of the Committee shared other sorts of beliefs as well. As was mentioned earlier in Chapter Four, the claim that the medical profession was patriarchal both in its structure and attitude/beliefs, is an uncontentious one. None of the members of the committee had any previous history of challenging any of the orthodoxies with regard to women. None of the members of the committee thought to seriously challenge the patriarchal approach to the screening programme, and significantly, the only members who did make any reference to the fact that the women in the target groups might not be significantly better off as a result of the screening programme were the female members of the committee, and their objections were couched in very mild terms, and did not appear in the Forrest Report, but only subsequently in letters to the *British Medical Journal*. We must also not forget that one of the characteristics of the medical profession (like many other institutions), is that it prefers to recruit and promote individuals who hold similar attitudes and values to the existing members. Those who openly challenge orthodoxies find it very hard to advance their career. As is well demonstrated by the Wendy Savage enquiry, and is also well documented elsewhere, (Hearn, 1989; Saffron, 1983). It therefore seems plausible, given both the highly conventional background of the members of the committee, plus the deeply patriarchal nature of the medical profession in general, that we should attribute patriarchal beliefs to the members of the Forrest committee in particular.

Another way to approach the problem of establishing the existence of patriarchal beliefs in the 'minds' of the members of the Forrest Committee would be to approach the matter in the same way that Pateman and Gilligan both do in their respective studies of elite discourses. That is an analysis of the texts involved. In this case the most easily available text is the Forrest Report itself.

The Forrest Report is 67 pages long (excluding appendices). And its language and tone is both 'scientific' and statistical. This perhaps is unsurprising since medical science, almost by its nature, is more concerned with population based research rather than the in depth analysis of individual cases. Science, as a whole, even the more 'human' sciences, has a preference for the kind of data that can be *quantified*, counted, and subjected to statistical analysis. But even taking this into account, one might expect some consideration of the individual woman when it comes to an assessment of, for example, the benefits of clinical examination of the woman's breasts as opposed to self examination of the breasts. The report states (p. 23), that clinical examination of the breasts (that is, the examination of the breasts by a doctor) is not effective, and should not be considered as a screening method since there is little or no hope that such a procedure could reduce mortality rates from the disease. Yet the Committee's recommendations are that it should be carried out at every screening appointment. This would be more advantageous than self examination of the breasts (which they also claim is ineffective, but for different reasons). This preference for clinical breast examination (CBE) over breast self examination (BSE) is interesting for a number of reasons. Despite research findings that women are actually much better than doctors at detecting very small lumps in their own breasts, when they *do* carry out self examination of the breasts, the Forrest committee report makes it clear that they have a strong preference for clinical rather than self examination of the breasts. This preference seems to be because women still persistently do not immediately consult their doctors when they discover a lump. Instead they may wait weeks or even months before they present with what is described in the Forrest Report as 'advanced disease' (p. 22). The members of the committee seem to be mystified by this response, and clearly regard it as irrational. But no serious consideration is given to the reasons *why* women might not do the 'rational' thing and go immediately to their doctors. One obvious line of explanation is that it is a gendered understanding of the 'rational', rather in the way that Gilligan suggested in Chapter Four. Women are well aware that the discovery of a lump in their breasts might signal the discovery of a cancer. And women are also very well aware of the possible consequences attendant upon such a discovery. If a woman is diagnosed as having cancer (rightly or wrongly) she immediately becomes identified as a 'patient', and the subsequent treatment options may be painful, disfiguring and traumatic. There is also evidence to suggest (as discussed in Chapter Two that earlier diagnosis does not necessarily mean an improved prognosis. Can a woman's reluctance to consult her doctor as soon as she discovers a lump really be regarded as such an irrational action? But in keeping with the 'depersonalised' approach of medical science, no one has so far though of interviewing women (or indeed doing any kind of research) to find out why women do not seem to conform to the medical professions expected pattern of behaviour.

Under the section entitled 'Costs to patients' (p. 55), the Forrest report mentions the possible psychological costs associated with the screening process, but clearly considers that if there is such a cost, it is negligible:

Although *in theory*, to estimate a value for such psychological

119

factors, no work has yet been carried out on this issue. Indeed, there is no hard evidence to say whether there is a net cost to be considered (p. 55).

Perhaps such 'hard evidence' may have helped the Forrest committee predict the low take up rate that occurred after the programme was implemented, since women themselves were clearly not willing to come forward to be screened in anything like the numbers necessary for the programme to succeed. It is also interesting to note that the issue of psychological cost was not considered important enough to require any research. Under the heading 'Benefits', the report mentions the hoped for reduction in mortality rates, and then goes on to consider the various 'production gains'. Here, the committee considers the 'intrinsic value' of extending life, and then goes on to consider the gains to society of an extended working life. The committee magnanimously admit that there may be some economic value, even in housework!

Housework, for example, has a value, even though it is not paid for (p. 56).

The assumptions that are being made here, hardly need highlighting. The determination to disregard the individual is also evident in the figures and statistics that the Forrest Report contains as evidence to support its recommendations. This may be even more surprising given the importance of the actions of individual women (in coming forward for screening) who are vital if the breast cancer screening programme was to be 'successful'.

Another approach to the attribution of patriarchal beliefs to the members of the Forrest Committee would be to approach their recommendations in terms of 'who benefits' rather in the way that Walby does. If this method is adopted, what is clear is that women in the target group (ie those aged between 50 and 65) stand to gain very little in terms of increased life expectancy, even if they are *correctly* diagnoses as having cancer of the breast. In addition to this are the rather large numbers of women who are wrongly diagnosed, or to put it another way are 'false positives'. These women do not only suffer psychological damage as a result of the anxiety undoubtedly generated by such a false diagnosis, but they also stand to suffer physical harm in the form of unnecessary surgery, biopsies and repeated exposure to additional mammograms and clinical examinations. On the other hand, it could be argued that the medical profession are in a position to make gains from the programme, not just in terms of increased funding and status, but also in terms of another area of medical intervention and control of women's lives. Which further reinforces the patriarchal power of the doctor.

2 What the model would predict

Given these initial assumptions about the selection and composition of the committee, what course of action would the revised Sabatier model predict that the Forrest Committee would take?

The first issue which we will look at concerns control of information. Sabatier suggests that within policy sub-systems, the elite discourse and the conflict between the advocacy coalitions leads to what he calls policy-oriented learning. The upshot of this is that knowledge about the issue area improves over time as each advocacy coalition produces research findings to support its position in the face of opposing claims and information from other groups. But we now have reason to think that this is a rather naive characterisation of the process of policy-oriented learning. Although Sabatier recognises the existence of dominant groups within the policy sub-system, but he doesn't seem to notice the possible distorting effects that this might have on the processes and products of policy oriented learning. The revised model would predict that, given the apparent consensus among the members of the dominant advocacy coalition, and given also their structurally strong position, they might try to manipulate or control the information flowing in and out of the policy system. This control of the knowledge or information might be regarded as having two separate strands, firstly, as mentioned before, the control of the information flowing in and out of the process of policy oriented learning, and secondly, the type of knowledge that is either 'allowed' or 'rejected' may change according to the changing power structure of the advocacy coalitions. It must also be noticed that the control of information operates at two levels, that is from 'expert to expert' and also from 'expert to non-expert'. At the first level, this simply means that within the elite discourse, the dominant group, or advocacy coalition are in a better structural position to exclude 'unwanted' information. In the case of breast cancer screening, this meant that the highly influential and powerful Forrest Committee were fairly successful at excluding the voices of opponents of the breast cancer screening programme such as Skrabanek, Roberts and Ellman. Importantly, various members of the Forrest Committee were able to publish, in highly regarded medical journals, their pro-screening views, whereas it was much more difficult for opponents, such as

Skrabanek to do the same. (In a personal interview, Petr Skrabanek confided that one editor of such a journal referred to his work as 'scurrilous' and refused to publish it).

At the second level, 'expert' to 'non-expert', we have a different situation. Having achieved a degree of structural dominance, a powerful advocacy coalition is then in a position to manipulate the information flowing through 'official' channels to the general public. In the case of breast cancer screening the model would predict that given the pre-disposition of the members of the Forrest Committee that the information that became 'officially' available to the 'woman on the street' would be strongly in favour of breast cancer screening. And this is precisely the case. In fact there was, and still is, despite recent developments, a powerful drive to get women to come forward for routine screening of their breasts. But the information leaflets that the women were offered, through GPs' surgeries, Family Planning Clinics, Community Health Councils and Well Woman Clinics did NOT contain any information regarding the problems of false positives or false negatives, or the 'real' costs and benefits relating to the procedure. The impropriety of not fully informing women about possible negative effects of the screening process is one which has attracted a little attention, but certainly not enough fuss has been made to encourage the producers of the information to rethink their approach. The importance of this type of information control must not be underestimated, because it gives the relatively uninformed general public an impression of medical consensus. Which suggests that there is no need to question the policy. Women, even now, at 'grass roots' level are largely unaware that the breast cancer screening programme carries with it any risks. Indeed, quite the opposite. The 'ideological pressure' that this generates makes it all the easier for the powerful advocacy coalitions to use 'public opinion' to their advantage.

Secondly, the model would predict that the Committee would *use* this control of information in order to favour policies which leave power in the hands of men, and keep women in a subordinate role. It would thus predict that given a choice between treatment which the patient can administer in her own home, and treatment which requires her to come to a clinic (the doctor's home ground), the Committee (and the medical profession in general) would opt for the latter. Given a choice between treatment which is low tech, and can be used and understood by the patient herself, and treatment which is high tech and cannot be used by the patient herself but only by the (usually male) doctor, the medical profession will go for the latter. This last point is especially relevant with respect to breast self examination, and clinical breast examination. There is plenty of evidence to suggest that women are very good at detecting even very small abnormalities in their breasts, if they look for them. Findings from the Nottingham BSE trials suggested that they were at least as good as doctors at finding lumps of less than 5cm. Yet there was considerable doubt that women were able to carry out breast self examination successfully. Despite various 'education' campaigns, GPs were advised to routinely (if possible) clinically examine the breasts of women who fell into any of the known 'high risk' groups, even if they were attending the doctors surgery concerning some other matter. This, coupled with the tendency to prefer hi tech solutions, is the link made by Oakley (among others) of technology and patriarchy. She notes that science and technology (a male preserve, especially in the 1900s) uses the mastery and possession of technology as a symbol of male control. The 'power' of science and technology remains in the hands of the male dominated medical profession, and out of the hands of the female patients. More abstractly then, the model would predict a preference on the part of the medical profession in general, and the Forrest Committee in particular, to 'go' for solutions that keep women passive, men active; women ignorant and men experts.

Thirdly, the model would lead us to expect that in assessing the pros and cons of various policy options, the Committee would be particularly insensitive to certain kinds of responses. For example, as Ehrenrich and English (1986) note, science, in general, has a predilection for *quantifiable* data. That is it prefers the sort of data that can be expressed numerically. An example of this kind of preference might be illustrated by the kinds of evidence seriously considered by the Forrest Committee concerning the usefulness of breast cancer screening. Womens' 'emotional' responses were not seriously taken into consideration, in that the emotional stresses and strains caused particularly by false positives, was not given any serious consideration by the Committee. Their prime focus of concern were quantifiable data, such as mortality rates. It is hard to quantify anxiety, therefore it tends to be ignored, and this is then justified on the basis of 'scientific objectivity'.

3 Matching the model with reality

When we turn from the model to the actual behaviour of the committee, we find significant confirmation of the predictions derived from the model. Firstly, in relation to control of information, we have found how (in Chapter Three) how the Committee was highly selective in relation to the information which it allowed into the policy area. It simply ignored, for example, some of the evidence from overseas trials which suggested that the proposed screening programme was not the best option. This was in spite of the fact that (as we saw in Chapter Two) this evidence met all the standard criteria for being 'good' evidence.

Nor was this the only evidence which was ignored. Only two members of the Forrest Committee were openly critical of the breast cancer screening programme. One of these, Dr Maureen Roberts voiced her concern at a number of meetings of the committee, but her opinions had been ignored. Petr Skrabanek, who had been a participating expert on the Forrest Committee, and Dr Austoker, who had been involved in the steering committee for the UK trial, both remarked to me in interviews that Dr Roberts had been increasingly concerned that the breast cancer screening programme was flawed and that it was not in women patients' interests to implement a national programme. After her death, the *British Medical Journal* published a posthumous letter from her which clearly stated her doubts about the wisdom of the programme. The main response to the letter came from Joslin Chamberlain, whose patronising tone prompted Dr Joan Austoker to remark in an interview that:

> Everyone thought that she [Dr Roberts] had become over emotional and subjective because she was suffering from breast cancer herself (Personal interview, 1993)

The other member of the Committee who voiced some disquiet about the breast cancer screening programme was Dr Ruth Ellman. Neither Roberts nor Ellman were completely hostile to the idea of screening for breast cancer, but both advised a more cautious approach. They argued that the problems associated with false positives and false negatives mentioned earlier, were unresolved, and that there were difficulties associated with the management of the disease once it had been correctly diagnosed. Both women believed subsequently that their opinions and advice had been ignored by the other members of the Committee. In the end, they felt that the only way in which they could make their voices heard was by writing to medical journals, such as the *British Medical Journal*.

Perhaps even more striking was the way in which the views of Petr Skrabanek were marginalised. Although he was on the list of participating experts, he alone among the participating experts was not required to attend any of the committee's meetings to give evidence, but was asked to submit his opinions in writing. During interview with me, he said that he thought that the committee had not bothered to read his papers, as he received no comments on them. He did in fact (in his words) 'gatecrash' a couple of meetings, where his reception had been 'frosty'.

There is one other respect in which the Committee's control of information (or better perhaps, *weighting* of information) needs to be noticed. As we saw in Chapter Two, the screening by mammography programme was 'inefficient' along two dimensions: missing cases which it 'should' have detected (false negatives), and falsely 'detecting' cases when the patient was in fact healthy (false positives). From an 'objective' point of view, the first group of cases matter much more. Failure to detect a condition for which further treatment may be available means (so supporters of the programme must believe) that a patient who could have been helped will not be helped, or at least will not be helped as quickly as she could have been. At the limit, it will mean (so supporters must believe) that a patient dies who could have been saved. By contrast, none of the false positives are women whose measurable condition will worsen as a consequence of the false diagnosis. None of them are women who will die because of that mistaken diagnosis. It would be 'natural' therefore to think that a high rate of false positives is not a major weakness in a screening programme.

But [and this is where patriarchal influences can be seen] this perception of the balance between false positive and false negatives reveals peculiarly male conceptions. What it ignores in arriving at this balance is the *psychological* stress on those women who are false positives. They are induced to believe that they may have a potentially life-threatening disease by the initial diagnosis; and they are then subjected to further medical procedures up to an including surgery, there was nothing *known* to be wrong with them in the first place! This stress, to which men are immune, is precisely the sort of factor that an underlying patriarchal outlook would minimise as women being over-reacting, being 'emotional', being 'subjective', and not 'looking at the facts'. The fact that the Committee could give so little weight to this problem of false positives is another instance of the way in which patriarchal attitudes influenced their handling of information. Indeed, as mentioned earlier, the psychological stress caused by the screening programme was an issue on which there was 'no hard evidence' (Forrest, 1986, p. 55) and which so far had not warranted any research at all.

This gives us, then, a major confirmation of the merits of our revised Sabatier model. The model predicts that the power relationships involved in a policy arena will result, not in the 'open' learning suggested by Sabatier, but rather in a purposeful control of information. Further, given the patriarchal nature of the committee, the model would predict that this control of information would be exercised in a patriarchal way. And that is precisely what we now find. Evidence against the patriarchal 'high tech' approach of screening by mammography is systematically marginalised. Its supporters are not invited onto the committee in the first place, nor invited to submit their evidence in person (Skrabanek); or have their fears dismissed because they are women, who, even though medically qualified, are still thought to be 'emotional' or 'subjective, or whose academic judgement is somehow clouded.

Let us consider, secondly, the prediction that the Committee would favour expensive high-tech solutions that keep power in the hands of the largely male doctors. It will be instructive here to compare the Committee's attitude to breast self-examination and to screening using mammography.

As was shown in Chapter Two, the evidence that self-examination of the breast was beneficial was rather thin. But we have also seen that the evidence supporting screening using mammography was also inconclusive. Why then abandon one ineffective method of screening for another (and much more expensive) ineffective screening method? When considering this question, we need to bear two points in mind: firstly, the preference of the medical profession for hi-tech procedures; and secondly, the nature of the doctor- patient relationship. In many ways, these two aspects are closely linked. Oakley (1982) has shown that *one* of the ways in which doctors in the past usurped the position of midwives was through the use of 'hi-tech' equipment. In that case, the crucial piece of equipment was forceps. The exact design of the instruments was kept secret from the female midwives who were not allowed to use them. Today, although the instruments have changed, the logic is the same. The use of highly specialised and highly technical equipment gives the doctor status and power, and this is true both within the profession and outside it. Highly technical branches of medicine are awarded higher status and attract more funding. Thus, brain surgery has a higher status than, for example, geriatrics. And the acquisition of technical equipment is almost always regarded as an 'improvement' in medical technique. The acquisition of new technical equipment also requires the acquisition of new skills on the part of the doctor, and this also brings with it enhanced status.

One of the 'side effects' of the increasing technology is the increasing passivity of the patient. This is also well-documented (Daly, 1984; Oakley, 1986) in the area of obstetrics, where women have their movements during labour restricted so that the doctor can attach various bits of monitoring equipment to both the woman and her unborn child. We can now see that the Forrest Committee's preference for screening by mammography fits into a larger pattern. Neither screening by mammography nor self-examination had a *very* impressive record of success; but there were other very significant differences between them. Breast self-examination was something that women could do for themselves. They had control of the whole process — *when* the examination was carried out, *how* it was done, *how long* it would last, *how often* it would be done, and so on. It is a corollary of this 'patient-power' that the role of the doctor was significantly reduced. (Of course, doctors would still have a major role to play for those women who reported symptoms but this would apply only to a minority of women as a whole.) By contrast, screening using mammography totally removed this control from the woman and placed it firmly back into the hands of the doctor. The examination had to take place outside the woman's own home in alien surroundings; it was done at a time to suit the timetable of the doctor; it was done using a technique which left the woman entirely passive, half naked in the presence of a team of radiologists and in a state of high anxiety and discomfort.

Once we highlight these differences between the two methods of screening, we can see how the Committee's firm line in favour of screening by mammography was necessarily opting for a solution which was in fact patriarchal. The revised model tells us that it was *because* it was patriarchal that it was favoured. It thus provides us with an explanation of the Committee's preference, a preference which as we saw in Chapter Three is hard to accommodate on any other model.

In short, the revised model renders explicable the actions of the Forrest Committee in a way that none of the other models achieves (it reaches parts that other models fail to reach?). Specifically, it copes with:

a. the apparent 'irrationality' the Forrest Committee displayed by ignoring crucial and 'respectable' evidence.
b. the Committee's preference for an expensive high tech solution over an inexpensive low tech solution
c. the importance of the structural relationship between the various advocacy coalitions, which influences both the process of policy oriented learning and the process and the manipulation of

information.

In addition to this, the revised model can also be used to explain the actions of the Government. When the minister for health announced the setting up of the Forrest Committee he had already decided who was going to chair the group. Perhaps predictably the chairman of the Working Group was male: (Sir Patrick Forrest), with, as we have already seen, a solidly orthodox medical background. Although there are generally speaking far fewer female consultants in the National Health Service than men, it would not have been impossible for Kenneth Clarke to appoint a woman as chairman of the Working Group. Jocelyn Chamberlain being the most obvious candidate. The selection of the remaining members of the committee was not the responsibility of the Secretary of State, but given, perhaps, the patriarchal preferences of the members of the Forrest Committee it is not surprising to find the gender balance of the committee biased in favour of males. The creation of the Working Group also occurred at a time when health ministers were under considerable pressure, via various 'interest groups' (as outlined in chapter one). Coupled with this pressure there was a growing awareness that in 'womens health issues' were not attracting sufficient Government resources. Just prior to the creation of the Forrest Committee, there had been considerable concern expressed in the media over the lack of funding for the cervical cancer screening programme, which had been so badly run that the call and recall system had failed to inform some women of positive findings, and women had died as a result. (Sharpe, 1987). In other area, for example ante natal screening, there was growing criticism against a barrage of tests which were carried out on a shoestring, and were of doubtful medical use. In *Screening in Health Care: Benefit or Bane*, Holland (1990) lists 26 tests which were routinely carried out at ante-natal clinics, of these only 15 had any medical evidence to support their use, and all of which were not carried out with optimum efficiency because of underfunding. It is also important to remember, as pointed out in chapter one, that there was a considerable amount of activity at the level of the backbenches to raise womens health issues in general, and breast screening in particular. For example, Edwina Curries outspoken support not only for breast cancer screening but for more and various government programmes of health promotion. Unlike the members of the Forrest Committee, it is difficult to do a textual analysis, but if we follow the example of Walby, and look at the policy outcome, in terms of a crude 'who wins' then it is possible to see that although there realm of expertise may have been different (i.e. politics rather than medicine), the policy outcome still demonstrated a patriarchal bias. One of the consequences of the decision to implement the national breast cancer screening service was that the Government gained a certain amount of political kudos; especially as they ring-fenced money to pay for the service, This also satisfied the explicitly stated wishes of the very powerful medical lobby, who had been pressing for action over breast cancer screening for some time. As in Walbys examples, those whom the policy was supposed to benefit the most, that is women in the target age group of 50-65 end up benefitting the least, as we have shown above.

4 Extension to other areas

But however good a theoretical model is at explaining *one* case, this is not in itself enough for us to be satisfied that it is a sound theoretical approach. It would need to be tested on a variety of case studies to strengthen its claim to being an explanatory framework. Obviously, the detailed provision of these further case studies lies beyond the limits of this thesis, but nevertheless it is incumbent on us to at least to suggest another fruitful area in which the model could be applied. One area that suggests itself is cervical cancer screening. This also has become a national screening service for women. If our framework is correct, we should be able to apply a similar analysis to this area of women's health. Very briefly, we would expect to discover that:

a. The programme was not in the interests of women
b. The preference of the medical profession was for a hi-tech solution which keeps the power in the hands of the medical profession, and
c. Certain sorts of information and evidence were ignored or disregarded.

We will briefly consider cervical screening programme to see if these predictions seem plausible.

Cervical cancer screening

Cancer of the neck of the womb is much less common than cancer of the breast. Mortality rates are less than a sixth of those from cancer of the breast. It also differs from cancer of the breast in that it is a more curable cancer because it spreads locally rather than from distant metastases.

Enthusiasm for screening began some twenty years ago following the publication of the results of trials in British Columbia (Smith, 1970). This enthusiasm was such as to lead doctors to forecast that the disease was going to be totally eradicated in the near future. However, the findings in British Columbia led others to examine what had been happening to mortality from this disease in other parts of the world, including some parts of Canada, where screening was unusual and where there were no organised programmes.

Screening for cervical cancer is based on the use of the cervical smear, or 'pap' test, named after Dr George Papanicolaou. It depends upon the doctor or nurse taking a scraping from the cervix with particular reference to the opening of the canal which leads from the vagina to the womb. The scrapings are then transferred to a microscope slide which is subsequently stained and examined for unusual cells. There are many possibilities for error during this process. The relevant part of the cervix may not be included in the smear, or the important cells may not be transferred to the slide; the examination of the slides has to be undertaken by doctors or technicians and they may either miss abnormal cells or describe normal cells as being abnormal. For all of these reasons, the incidence of false negatives is very high. The other major problem with the test is that although the prevalence of this cancer is low, many women will have smears which are reported as being abnormal, and these cells will be assumed to be suspicious and possibly pre-cancerous.

It is well established that these cells disappear if left alone, yet their existence, at the very least, creates anxiety in the woman who has been screened and often leads to colposcopy, and biopsy, and sometimes even to hysterectomy to be 'on the safe side'. These 'abnormalities' are very much more common than the disease, and this has led Alwyn Smith, a past president of the Faculty of Community Medicine to state:

It is absurd to conduct a screening test in such a way that nearly forty women are referred for an expensive and possibly hazardous procedure for every one who is at risk of developing serious disease (Champion et al, 1988)

In England and Wales, according to a *Lancet* editorial (1985), forty thousand smears and two hundred excision biopsies were performed for each cervical cancer death thought to have been prevented.

Although the exact cause of cervical cancer is unknown, there is a link between a woman's sexual activity and the disease. And it is this that deserves a little of our attention, given the context of this discussion. The terms sexual activity, promiscuity, marital stability, coitus at an early age, and prostitution are all bandied about in medical journals as defining the type of woman likely to get cervical cancer. Most of these terms are ambiguous and are rarely clearly explained. In *Cervical Cancer — The Politics Of Prevention*, Lisa Saffron (1983), points to the patriarchal attitudes expressed by the medical profession in the elite discourses on the subject of cervical cancer. She notes:

A double standard of morality is seen in nearly all the writings on cervical cancer. Very few studies asked about the man's sexual activity. One that did found that women whose husbands had fifteen or more sexual partners outside marriage were eight times more likely to get cervical cancer, even though the women themselves were monogamous. The interesting thing about the study is the tact with which the men were interviewed. To avoid arousing feelings of responsibility or guilt, the men were not told that the interviewer had anything to do with their wife's illness (1983, p. 45)

The doctors were not so delicate with the feelings of the women who contract the disease. An anonymous letter printed in *The Guardian* on the 7th June, 1982, reported a woman's experience after having had a cone biopsy. She remarked:

I was told by the gynaecologist that my cancer was the result of my promiscuity. When I asked if it were likely that the cancer would return, he said it was unlikely provided I behaved myself and didn't sleep with my boyfriend.

This particular woman then relates how she had then counted up the number of male partners she had had in the last ten years and the grand total was six.

Once a woman has been diagnosed as having cancer of the cervix the treatments also seem to reflect patriarchal attitudes. Saffron points out:

It is the nature of Western medicine to start with the most dramatic measure, to use a sledgehammer to crack a nut. Coupled with a contempt for women's bodies, our reproductive organs don't stand a chance. The rule of thumb seems to be that there is no cervix so healthy that it isn't better treated and no testis so diseased that it isn't better left intact. Men's reproductive organs simply do not get the kind of attention that women's do (1983, p. 47)

Jean Robinson asks:

Isn't it time for women to ask why the medical profession advocated a policy of screening but denied women information that would allow them to chose primary prevention (i.e. condoms or celibacy)? Why also, did the information that women's promiscuity 'caused' cervical cancer get through to women, whereas the risk of male promiscuity did not? (1985, p. 51)

She concluded:

The fact is that the cervical cancer screening programme has been based on a view of women as passive patients. To be urged to come for smears, rebuked as irresponsible if they do not, scolded like naughty children if they have the disease that screening was meant to detect, and then sent home to go on living with the same promiscuous man or to go on taking the pill. A view of women as active controllers of their own bodies would suggest a different policy and would go for primary prevention (1985, p. 51).

What Robinson and Saffron are both suggesting is that as it stands, the cervical cancer screening service seems to be riddled with the kinds of attitudes that might be predicted from the discussion of patriarchal beliefs in the medical profession in Chapter Four. In particular, the medical profession seems to have defined this disease as being the woman's 'fault' and to have studiously ignored the evidence that the male half of the population held some responsibility for the spread of the disease. There has not been any serious consideration of the screening of men to find out if they are 'carriers', nor has there been any attempt to inform women of the effect that male 'promiscuity' may have on their chances of developing the disease. Instead, the medical profession have opted for a course of action which is the most interventionist and possibly the least effective. Instead of being advised to use condoms, women are subjected to biopsies and colposcopies.

The pattern that was observed, then, in the case of breast cancer screening seems not to be an isolated blindspot. But perhaps the pattern that is being observed is simply one that happens when the procedures and treatments are in those areas which deal exclusively with women. In order to test this challenge, it would be necessary to look at some examples of medical procedures which were common to both men and women to see if there were any differences in the way men and women were treated. Such areas might include the treatment of ischemic heart disease or hip replacement operations. In both of these examples, there is evidence which suggests that the treatment of women receives a lower priority than that of men (Clarke and Grey et al., 1994). If these were to be taken as case studies, then they would clearly need to be examined in detail, but superficially at least, there is reason to believe that the cases of breast cancer and cervical cancer screening are not exceptional.

5 Conclusion

At the beginning of the thesis, we asked the question, how do we explain the decision to implement a national programme of breast cancer screening? It quickly becomes apparent, on close examination of the medical evidence, that breast cancer screening is not the magic solution that many have claimed that it is. What remained for us to puzzle out was that, given this state of affairs, how could such a piece of institutional decision making be explained and understood? In search of the answer we turned first of all to the various types of rational actor approaches. This seemed the most logical place to start, since it is assumed by most, that medical science should, at least in some sense of the word, be rational. But however hard we tried, the rational action models seemed to be incapable of fully explaining the actions of the Forrest Committee, and even Sabatiers' model, though the most promising of all, was unsatisfactory. This must in part be blamed on the difficulties that each of the models had in defining exactly what is meant by 'rational' in the context of political decision making. Simple RA models have the attraction of being elegantly simple, but application of these turn out to be extremely difficult. The problem being that the way human beings behave in the 'real world' is rarely observably 'rational' in the way that RA models would have us believe. Unless we invent a new way of either conceptualising what is rational, or place the 'rational' into a different kind of context we seem to be faced with models that simply do not seem to 'fit' the 'facts'. One way of doing this was suggested by Sabatier, and involved the recognition of the role played by beliefs in the process of policy making. This seemed to offer a more satisfactory approach because some consideration of actors' beliefs seemed necessary if we were to place their actions into any kind of 'rational' context. But even this left us with problems. One of these problems is associated with establishing what peoples beliefs actually are. Especially if these beliefs are what might be called 'deep core' beliefs. As was discussed in

Chapter Three, both inferring what people believe from their actions and asking individuals to openly state what their beliefs are, is problematic for a variety of reasons. Nonetheless, we feel that this is a vital component if we are to understand any decision making process. This is because beliefs might be seen as forming a kind of 'baseline' or 'paradigm' from which policy options are chosen. For example: although in the UK we have a variety of political parties, pressure groups, and trades unions, all of these (or at least all of the 'respectable' ones) have a general commitment to capitalism. This may be viewed as a 'political paradigm' based on an underlying belief that capitalism is better than any other economic system. This is not a belief that needs to be constantly rehearsed in public, but it is clearly to be observed in the kinds of discourses and policies that emerge from the political machine. But it is not only the political and economic elite who believe in capitalism, no serious challenge to the economic order has so far emerged from the workforce. This creates a kind of ideological or political power 'gradient' against which radical change, or even fairly moderate change is extremely difficult. Unless this 'pressure' that beliefs or ideas create is recognised, it would seem that any deeper understanding of the decision making processes is difficult to achieve. In order to rectify some of the weaknesses of the previously discussed models, a new model has been suggested, and applied to the case study of breast cancer screening. This new model has the advantage of building on the previous ones and making them sensitive to the issues surrounding power and gender. Importantly, it recognises the role of entrenched, and often largely unexpressed, belief systems of the policy makers. All policy makers have beliefs, and these beliefs must influence both their actions and their policy preferences, but, as mentioned earlier, the beliefs of the individual must have some degree of congruity with the prevailing 'paradigm' this is what Sabatier calls the 'glue' of politics, but an appeal purely to the belief systems of the actors is not enough. It needs to be placed within the context of a power structure, and this is precisely what the new model allows us to do. The model may not be perfect, but it at least gives us an insight that the other models do not seem to offer. That is to say, it places this 'ideological pressure' into a power structure. For the purposes of this thesis we are not concerned so much with the consensus over the benefits of capitalism, instead our focus has been on the relative positions of men and women, and the beliefs and power structures that maintain that particular status quo. In other words we are concerned with patriarchal beliefs and power structures. What has clearly been shown is that patriarchal beliefs (and structures) are

134

endemic within the institution of medicine. But these beliefs are not peculiar to medicine. One does not need to probe very deeply to find such beliefs apparent in almost every institution of the state, and almost every business institution. We should therefore not be surprised if we see the government endorsing a policy which reflects patriarchal values and beliefs, any more than we would be surprised if they were advocating broadly capitalist policies. An application of our new model to the governments decision to implement the recommendations of the Forrest Committee could be approached in exactly the same way as the previously mentioned RA models. That is to say that it has some predictive power. The model would predict that they would prefer a policy option which maintained the patriarchal status quo, either in 'ideological' terms or in terms of the power structure. Some feminist writers would claim that in terms of entrenched patriarchal beliefs and structures, the various institutions of the state stand head and shoulders above the rest. Given this 'paradigm', it would be very surprising to see any kind of radical policy which leaned towards the empowerment of women. What we might expect to see, are policies which *seem* to serve the interests of women, but which in fact, do not. (Walby, 1990) None of the previously examined models, can really cope with the apparent mismatch between policy 'outcome' and policy 'intent' in the way that this new model can. Whatever the policy, and whatever the institution, policies and policy making has to be understood as taking place within this all pervading atmosphere of patriarchal beliefs. Our new model also explains why any radical change in the relative position of women in society in general is so hard to achieve. The ideological and political 'gradient' created by patriarchy seems all pervading, and it is significant that even political science has so far failed to observe that there is a 'gender issue' which needed to be addressed, at least as far as models of decision making is concerned. Some attempt at correcting this state of affairs has been attempted here, by focusing on one particular case study, but, as was suggested earlier, other areas of investigation are possible, both within health policy and outside it. The real test of any model of decision making is not just that it explain *one* case, but that it has a wider application. And that will be our next challenge.

References

Champion, J., Brown, J. R., McCance, D. J., et al.; (1988); 'Psychosexual Trauma of an Abnormal Cervical Smear', *British Journal of*

Obstetrics and Gynaecology, vol 95, pp. 175-181.

Editorial (1985); 'Cancer of the Cervix — Death by Incompetence', *The Lancet*, vol 11, pp. 363-364.

Hearn, J., Shepperd, D., Burrell, G., (eds); (1989); *The Sexuality of Organisations*, Sage, London.

Oakley, A; (1986); *The Captured Womb*, Basil Blackwell, London.

Robinson, J; (1985); 'Cervical Cancer - Doctors Hide the Truth', in *Womens Health — A Spare Rib Reader*, Pandora, London.

Saffron, L; (1983); 'Cervical Cancer, The Politics of Prevention', in *Womens Health: A Spare Rib Reader*, Pandora, London.

Skrabanek, P; (1988); 'Cervical Cancer Screening: A Time for Reappraisal', *Canadian Journal of Public Health*, Vol 79, pp. 80-9.

Skrabanek, P; (1988); *Follies and Fallacies in Medicine*, Paragon Press, Glasgow.

Appendix 1

Edited conclusions and recommendations of the Forrest
Committee Report

Chapter Four: Basic screening methods

On the information currently available, mammography alone is the
preferred option for basic screening. Unlike clinical examination and
BSE used alsone it is of proven effectiveness in reducing breast cancer
mortality among women aged 50 and over. Clinical examination and
BSE detect fewer of the early tumours for which treatment may have
the most effect on survival. Mammography is acceptable to women. Its
sensitivity is considerably greater than that of clinical examination and
its specificity in recalling women for further investigation is also high.
Any carcinogenic risk arising from its radiation is minute in relation to
its potential benefits in women aged 50 and over. It carries a potential
disadvantage of detecting early lesions that may never prove life
threatening and would not mormally present for treatment, but this is
mainly limited to the initial prevelence screen, and is of less
importance in subsequent screens.

   Any benefit resulting from combined as opposed to single method
screening must arise from the extra sensitivity gained by using two (or
more) tests as opposed to one. This is difficult to assess. Twenty years ago
the HIP New York study 42 per cent of screen detected cases would have
been missed if only mammography had been used. Since then
mammographic techniques have improved substantially so that in
current studies using both clinical examination and mammography only
5-10 per cent of cases wouls be missed if only mammography were used.
However, the objective of screening is not case detection but improved
prognosis for cases detected at screening. The marginal cost of adding
clinical examination to mammography is high in terms of cancers
detected, but is unknown in terms of life years gained.

   The extent of any gain from BSE education in the screening
proceedure is also difficult to assess because the method of assessing

137

sensitivity assumes that any cancers diagnosed in the twelve months following a screen are 'false negatives' to that screen. However, these cases may be 'true positives' to the BSE education component of combined-method screening because the woman has detected them herself earlier than if she had not been encouraged to perform BSE. Hence a screening programme incorporation BSE education may appear to have a high number of interval cases bacause it increases the number of cancers discovered by the woman herself. This programme will appear to have a low sensitivity but it may still achieve a high proportion of cancers diagnosed at an early stage — and a greater reduction in mortality — than programmes without BSE education. The additional benefit to be gained by adding BSE education to mammography would probably be greater the longer the interval between mammographic screens.

> *High quality single mdieo-lateral oblique view mammography has been shown to be an effective method in reducing mortality from breast cancer and we conclude that initially this is the preferred option for the development of mass population screening.*
> *There is no evidence that clinical examination or breast self examination is effective when used alsone. These methods have some value when used in combination with mammography but their contribution required further assessment.*
> *The remainder of our report assumes that single view mammography is the method to be employed for basic screening in a mass population screening programme.* (emphasis in original, pp. 24-25)

Chapter Five: Basic screening selection and frequency

Selection by age

There is clear evidence that women aged 50 and over are likely to benefit from screening. Further evidence on the effectiveness of screening women under 50 is required: studies are continuing in the UK, Canada and Sweden. Women up to age 65 should be positively encouraged to be regularly screened, but after this age screening should be provided only for those who request it.

Selection by other risk factors

The use of risk factors other than age to identify women in the general population who should be screened is not practicable at present. This is not to say that individual patients who have sought advice about breast problems and who have one or more recognised risk factors should not be investigated, but it is for the responisible clinician to decide. For a population screening programme the only feasible criterion for selection at present is initially to limit screeninf to women aged 50 and over.

Frequency

There is clearly a need for further research into the costs and benefits of screening at different intervals to identify an optimum screening interval. The Swedish study shows a substantial benefit in women aged 50 and over with a screening interval of nearly three years. Until the optimum frequency has been determind we suggest that the interval should be three years.

Conclusions

The effectiveness of screening has so far been demonstrated only for women aged 50 and over. In view of the poor response rates there is insufficient benefit to be gained by actively offering screening to women aged 65 and over. The priority of any screening programme should therefore be given to offering an initial screen to as many women as possible aged between 50-64 years of age. This does not exclude making screening available on demand to older women.

The use of risk factors other than age to identify women in the general population who should be screened is not practicable at present.

There is insufficient evidence on the optimum frequency for routine repeated screening and its determination must have high priority for immdediate research. As a starting point for the screening programme we suggest an interval of three years but this must be kept under review.

Chapter Six: Assessment, biopsy and treatment

Recall for additional films

In chapter Four we concluded that mammography alone was the preferred option for the basic screen. We also concluded that high quality single view mammography could be effective. When only a single view is used, it is estimated that up to 10 per cent of the women screened might be required to have an additional cranial-caudal view and a repeat medio-lateral view to define the nature of an artefact or composite shadow. This would be done at a subsequent visit to the basic screening unit.

Assessment

When a basic screening result is confirmed as abnormal it must be assessed. In addition any women who report symptoms e.g. breast lump or distortion, at the basic screen must be referred for assessment.

In Chapter Three the following techniques which were available for the assessment of screen detected abnormalities:

Clinical examination
Sophisticated mammography
Ultrasonography
Fine needle aspiration
Fine needle aspiration cytology
Clinical examination

All women referred for assessment must have a clinical examination of the breast to establish whether palpable leisions are present in the light of the mammographic findings. It is essential that this examination is carried out by a clinician experienced in the signs and symptoms of early breast cancer.

Sophisticated mammography

For suspicios leisions, additional mammographic study is necessary using machines not only with moving grids, but also with facilities for magnification views and needle localisation techniques. These units are more sophisticated that the simpler machines appropriate forbasic screening and are therefore more expensive. Such machines are likely to be located in a hospital, where they will also be used for the invstigation of symptomatic patients.

Ultrasonography

Ultrasound cannot at present be used as a basic screening technique because it fails to detect the majority of solid impalpable leisions.

However, when used to compliment mammography it is a valuable assessment technique. e.g. to confirm the cystic nature of an impalpable leision or to help in guided-needle biopsy or sampling. A simple machine is considered satsfactory.

Fine needle aspiration

This is a valuable method of differentiating cystic from solid lesions. This applies not only to palpable lesions but also to impalpable small mammographic opacities. For the aspiration of these small lesions ultrasonic guidance is helpful.

Fine needle aspiration cytology

This technique is used to examine cells aspirated from suspicious solid lesions, whether palpable or inpalpable. Its place in differentiating benign from malignant lesions is now established.

Specialist assessment teams

In Chapter Three we discussed two possible routes by which a screen detected abnormality could be referred for assessment. The basic screening unit would refer a woman either to her general practitioner or, with the prior consent of the general practitioner, direct to a specialist assessment team. If the general practitioner chooses to arrange the assessment, her or she may decide to refer the woman to a surgeon of her choice. If the surgeon does not have access to the specialised assessment techniques this may lead to a high biopsy rate together with a higher ratio of benign to malignant biopsies.

In existing UK trial centres almost all general practitioner have preferred that the screening team refer women with suspected abnormalities directly to a specialist assessment team, in which event the general practitioner must be kept informed. Some general practitioners may wish to be consulted if an excision biopsy is recommended, others are willing to accept the advice of the assessment team.

The assessment team consists of a clinician, a radiologist and a pathologist all trained in the diagnosis of breast disease, supported by a radiographer, a nurse and a receptionist. The clinician not only has to be responsible for clinically examining the breasts and possibly performing fine needle aspiration, but also has an important role, in consultation with colleagues in co-ordinating the results of the investigations and in making the decision as to whether the lesion merits biopsy. The clinician must also discuss the implications with the woman concerned. In centres with a surgeon having a special interest in breast disease it is likely that the sugeon will wish to be associated with the assessment procedure. However the surgeon may have insufficient time to participate actively, and responsibility for co-ordinating the assessment proceedure will fall to another clinician who may or may not be a member of the surgeon's team. It is unlikely that the pattern will be the same in each centre. In Edinburgh and Guildford the clinician in charge of the basic screening unit has assumed this role.

The advantages of an assessment team are as follows:

The continuing sharing of experience and review of cases within a multidisciplinary team;
Immediate co-ordination of clinical, radiological and pathological findings to reach a decision on the need for a biopsy or treatment as soon as possible;
Fine needle aspiration under mammographic and ultrasonic control may be done at the first attendance and immdediate cytological reporting may be available.

Hospital or community based clinic

The assessment techniques may be carried out either in hospital or in a clinic in the community. The choice will depend on local circumstances, for example population density. If the choice is a hospital, it is desirable that women are seen sepaerately from those attending a diagnostic clinic for symptomatic women.

Biopsy

An open or excision biopsy may be carried out either under local or general anaesthesia. X-ray localisation techniques are rquired for the impalpable lesion, removal of which must be conbfirmed by specimen radiology best carried out using dedicated apparatus. Similarly, the histological examination of these specimens requires radiological as well as histological facilities. We consider there is no place for the examination of these lesions by frozen section technology.

Treatment

Screening is not likely to lead to a significant increase in the numbers of breast cancers treated. During the initial (prevalence) screen there will be an increase in the numbers treated, but this may eventually be compensated by a subsequent reduction in the normally expected incidence. The only potential source of a general increase in the numbers treated would seem to be from cancers that wouls not otherwise be detected because death from another cause may occur prior to symptoms arising. The detection of a larger number of in-situ cancers and small invasive cancers will favour the use of conservation techniques and this may increase cetain aspects of threaputic workload; for example radiotherapy.

Conclusions

The assessment of screen detected abnormalities requires specialised techniques. These techniques are best carried out by a skilled multidisciplinary team, either within a hospital or a clinic in the community. This team should consist of a clinician, a radiologist and a pathologist all trained in the diagnosis of breast diseas, supported by a radiographer, a nurse and a receptionist. The availablity of such teams is an essential prerequisite of a screening service for breast cancer.

Biopsies of impalpable screen detected abnormalities should be performed, wherever possible, by a specialised breast team experienced in the surgical, radiological and pathological skills necessary for localisation techniques.

During the prevalence screen there will be an increase in the numbers to be biopsied and treated for breast cancer. While this may initially increas the owrkload there should be a subsequent reduction to the normally expected incidence. The detection of larger numbers of in-situ cancers ans small invasive cancers will favour the use of conservation techniques and this may increase certain aspects of the theraputic workload; for example, radiotherapy.

Chapter Seven: Organisation of a screening service

Introduction

The evidence reviewed in the previous chapters leads us to conclude that a screening service for women aged 50 to 64 using mammography for the basic screen is initially the preferred option. Although evidence on the best interval between repeat screens is still unclear we suggested in Chapter Five that a three year interval may be used during the development of a screening programme but that research is required to determine the optimum interval. This chapter suggests how such a screening service may be organised in the United Kingdom, and is based on the experience of the Edinburgh and Guildford screening programmes which form part of the UK Trial of Early Detection of Breast Cancer. It is only as illustration of how a screening programme may be organised, we accept that other arrangements may be preferred in the light of local circumstances.

Indentifying women to be screened

The eligable population can be best identified from the registers of women on genral practitioner's lists. These lists are held by Family Practitioner Committees (FPC) in England and Wales and by Area Health Boards in Scotland and give womens' names and addresses of their general practitioners. Although these registers are known to have a number of inaccuracies (up to twenty per cent of addressess may be inaccurate) they are the only source of the information required.

Invitations to be screened

Systems for inviting women to be screened for cervical cancer have already been developed and can be adapted and enhanced for breast cancer screening. In England and Wales the FPC will send to each general practitioner, at regular intervals, a list of those eligible for screening. The general practitioner will delete the names of women for whom screening is contraindicated (e.g. because of illness), and return the list to the FPC. A computerised invitation letter will be sent, normally under the name of the general practitioner. The form of it will be for local decision. A reminder letter may be required for women who do not respond.

Non-invited women

Some women outside the invited age group for screening will wish to be screened. Women aged 65 and over should be allowed to attend for screening but need not be recalled routinely. As the evidence that women younger than 50 benefit from screening is uncertain, we suggest that they should consult their general practitioner who, if he or she considers tham at increased risk, may consult with the screening service.

Basic screening stage: taking mammograms

Clinical responsibility for individual women being screened will be taken by a doctor experienced in the clinical aspects of breast cancer screening, and who may be a consultant radiologist. The doctor will not need to be present at the screening clinics. At every screening attendence each woman will complete a short questionnaire. Essential information includes date of birth, presence in either breast of a lump or distortion, and past surgery with position of scars recorded. These data will be entered into a computerised record system. Mammography will be performed by a specially trained radiographer. Following mammography, the woman will be told how she can obtain the results of her test. Immediate processing of the films and processing of the films and assessment of their adequecy by experienced radiographers is unecessary and reduces the throughput of women. Films may be transported to a central processing unit.

Reading mammograms

The purpose of basic screening is not to make a diagnosis but to separate the women into those who need further investigation and those who do not. Reading the basic screening mammograms must be the resposibility of the consultant radiologist, although the task can be devolved. Where reading a film is devolved to a non-radiologist they will be trained to refer all films that are not obviously negative to the radiologist. The radiologist will then decide how to classify the difficult or suspicious films.

The reading of the mammograms will separate women into three groups: those with inadequate films for making a decision, those with positive findings requiring assessment, and those with negative findings.

Notification of results

The doctor with clinical responsibility for screening women will also be responsible for notifying both the woman concerned and her general practitioner of the result. Where a woman is found to have a mammographic abnormality or where she reports the presence of a breast lump or distortion, assessment is required. Depending on the prior wishes of the general practitioner the woman will be referred by the doctor responsible either to the general practitioner or directly to the specialist assessment team.

The location of the basic screening unit

A basic screening unit may be static or mobile, and according to local circumstances may be sited either within a community health clinic or hospital. Hospital based units should be seperate from the hospital diagnostic x-ray unit department because the organisation of a screening clinic requires a rapid throughput of well women with very different expectations from the patients undergoing diagnostic x-ray investigation.

Assessment and biopsy

A medical member of the [assessment] team must be resposible for the following: co-ordinating the results of further investigations, reaching a decision on the need for biopsy or treatment and making the appropriate arrangements, and notifying the woman, general practitioner and the central screening office.

Screening records system

A screening record system should be developed to fulfill the following functions: (i) identification and recall of eligible women for screening, (ii) attendance for screening and results; (iii) monitoring the screening process; (iv) monitoring effectiveness. The system should be computerised with links to the appropriate population register.

Identification, invitation and recall. The FPC registers in England and Wales, and their equivalents in Scotland and Northern Ireland, form the basis for identification of eligible women and, with computerisation, enable an invitation system to be implemented with the genral practitioners consent.

Attendance for screening and results. A simple basic record is required giving identification particulars, date of attendance, present breast symptoms and past breast surgery. This record will accompany the mammographic films to the radiologist who will be responsible for adding the screening opinion in terms of routine recall, repeat film or referral for treatment.

Monitoring the screening process. Linkage to local pathology registers and cancer registries is desirable so that the diagnosis of breast cancer can be added to the relavent womans record, if this is not already known.

Monitoring the effectiveness of screening. This can be done approximately by examining trends in age specific breast cancer mortality available from routine statistics. However, linkage of mortality data to screening will enable a more precise and useful method of monitoring effectiveness, in that deaths from breast cancer can be categorised into those among women diagnosed by screening, those in interval cases, those in women who refused screening, and those non-invited women.

Quality control of mammography

To achieve the high standards required in mammographic screening service, meticulous quality control is mandatory. The consultant radiologist together with the medical physicist and radiographers, in accordance with normal practice, will be responsible for ensuring quality control in each basic screening unit.

Radiation protection and monitoring

The radiation protection of both staff and those who are to be screened will need to be secured and monitored in accordance with ionising radiations regulations (1985) and the ionising radiations (protection of persons undergoing medical examination or treatment) regulations.

Management

The data presented earlier suggests that basic screening units will serve populations generally larger than those of English district health authorities, or their equivalents in other UK countries, and that the specialist assessment teams may serve an even larger catchment area. It is essential that every health authority or group of health authorities should designate one person with responsibility for the organisation, planning and epidemiological monitoring of the breast cancer screening programme for a defined population of women. Ideally this person will be a specialist in community medicine, who will undertake the responibilty in addition to other duties in preventive medical care.

Conclusions

While no one organisational solution for a screening programme is necessarily right for each health authority, a plan for a screening programme should include the following:

1 Women in the target group should be sent a personal invitation from their general practitioner.

2 Arrangements for recording results at the basic screen must include a fail-safe mechanism, to ensure that action is taken on all positive reults.
3 Every basic screening unit must have access to a specialist team for the assessment of screen detected abnormalities.
4 A screening record system should be developed to identify, invite and recall women eligible for screening; to record attendance for screening and results; and to monitor the screening process and its effectiveness.
5 There should be adequate arrangements for quality control both within and between centres so that an acceptable standard of mammography can be maintained.
6 A designated person should be responsible for managing each local screening service. The person chosen would have manegerial ability and is likely to have experience in community or preventive health care, although the radiological aspects must be the responibility of a consultant radiologist. Setting up a breast screening service will require substantial manegerial effort.

We can see considerable advantage in forming central bodies to advise Health Departments on the introduction of breast cance screening programmes, to monitor their effectiveness and efficiency and to keep their progress under review. Such bodies might also advise their Health Departments on future policy.

Chapter Eight: Service requirements

Conclusions

The manpower implications for radiologists and radiographers are critical to the introduction of a screening programme. No centre should undertake screening without having a high level of expertise in mammography in order to minimise false-negative and false-positive findings.

The training of staff and the maintenance of quality is important in all relavent discaplines and for all stage of the screening process. The required expertise will need to be spread progressvely from existing centres.

A basic screening unit, screening 12,000 women a year, could serve a population of some 41,500 women aged 50-64 within a total population of nearly half a million. This implies a requirement for around 120 basic units throughout the UK. This fewer than the number of districts and boards in the UK (219). In view of the shortage of trained staff and the cost equipment, it would be more cost effective. if practicable, for each basic screening unit to serve the maximum population rather than to have one for each district or board.

Specialist assessment teams should be developed in those districts or boards with the necessary expertise in breast cancer diagnosis, each team working a sufficient number of sessions to provide for referrals from 1-3 basic screening units.

An established UK breast cancer screening programme with 120 basic screening units will require some 930 Whole Time Equivalent staff including about 40 radiologists and some 200 radiographers.

In practice, both biopsies and treatment will increasingly be concentrated on a relatively small number of surgeons and supporting assessment teams, so that any overall increase in workload will not be evenly distributed.

Training of radiologists and radiographers will have some manpower implications in the development phase of a screening programme, but these should be negligible in the long term.

Introducing a screening programme will initially require substantial capital investment in equipment and buildings. A mobile unit may, in some circumstances, be the preferred option for basic screening.

Chapter Nine: Economic appraisal

The estimates for cost per life-year or cost per QALY gained for breast cancer screening are not dissimilar to other health service activities currently undertaken. It is possible that expansion of other services may offer higher returns on resources spent.

We estimate that the annual revenue cost to the NHS in the UK for running a screening service, based on the Edinburgh experience and with the parameters we suggest, is about £18 million (1985-86 prices). The capital cost is likely to be at most £31 million (1985-86 prices). More frequent screening or extending the service to a much wider range would require an increase in the number of basic units and, therefore, costs would increase pro rata.

Appendix 2

Brief biographical information on Forrest Committee members

Professor Sir Patrick Forrest

Held the Chair of Surgery at the Welsh National School of Medicine for nine years before moving to Edinburgh to take up the post of Professor of Clinical Surgery at Edinburgh University. As well as being the Chairman of the Working Group on breast cancer screening (and having a keen and active interest in breast cancer), he was also a member of the Breast Cancer Research Subcommittee and the Scottish Advisory Committee on breast screening. He was a member of Cancer Research Campaign and of the Royal College of Surgeons of Edinburgh.

Relevant publications

Aitkin, R., Forrest, A. P. M., et al., (1988); 'Radiology and Breast Cancer', vol 55, pp. 13-20.
Anderson, E. D. C., Forrest, A. P. M., et al., (1989), 'Response to Endocrine Manipulation and Oestrogen Receptor Concentration in Large Operable Primary Breast Cancer', *British Journal of Cancer*, vol 60, pp. 223-6
Anderson, T. J., Forrest, A. P. M., et al., (1983); 'Multi Focal Cancers in a Breast Screening Programme' Third European Organisation for Research and Treatment of Cancer, Breast Cancer Working Conference, Amsterdam.
Dean, C., Forrest, A. P. M., et al., (1983); 'Effect of Immediate Breast Reconstruction on Psychological Morbidity After Mastectomy', *The Lancet*, vol 1, pp. 459-62.
Forrest, A. P. M, (1955); 'Pituitary Radon Implant for Breast Cancer', *The Lancet*, vo 11, pp. 1054-5.
Forrest, A. P. M., (1986); 'A Human Tumour Model', *The Lancet*, vol 2, pp. 840-2.

Forrest, A. P. M., (1988); The Welbeck Memorial Lecture 1988, 'Radiology and Breast Cancer', *Radiology Today*, vol 55, pp. 13-20.

Forrest, A. P. M., (1989); 'Endocrine Management of Breast Cancer' in *Oestrogen and Human Breast Cancer*, Beck,J (ed), Proc. Royal Society of Education Board, vol 94, pp. 1-10.

Forrest, A. P. M, (1989); 'Lister Oration: Breast Cancer 121 Years On', *Journal of the Royal College of Surgery*, vol 34, pp. 239-48.

Forrest, A. P. M., (1989); 'The Surgeon's Role In Breast Screening', *World Journal of Surgery*, vol 13, pp. 19-24.

Forrest, A. P. M., Kunkler, P. B., (1968); 'Breast Cancer Management of the Early Case' *Hospital Medicine*, January, pp. 239-407.

Forrest, A. P. M., Blair, D. W., et al. (1958); 'Screw Implantation of the Pituitary with Yttruim 90' *The Lancet*, vol 2, pp. 192-3.

Forrest, A. P. M., Hawkins, R, A., Miller, W, R., (1989); 'Breast' in Jameson and Kay's *Textbook of Surgical Physiology*, Churchill and Livingstone, Edinburgh, pp. 85-94.

Furnival, I., Stewart, H., Forrest, A. P. M., et al., (1970); 'Accuracy of Screening Methods for the Diagnosis of Breast Disease', *British Medical Journal*, vol 4, pp. 461-3.

Macay, J., Forrest, A. P. M., et al., (1988); 'Allelle Loss on Short Arm of Chromosome 17 in Breast Cancers', *The Lancet*, vo l2, pp. 1384-6.

MacFayden, I., Forrest, A. P. M. (1976); 'Plasma Steroid Levels in Women with Breast Cancer', *The Lancet*, vol 1, pp. 1100-2.

Roberts, M., Alexander, F., Anderson, T., Forrest, A, P, M., (1984); 'The Edinburgh Randomised Trial of Screening for Breast Cancer: Description of Method', *British Journal of Cancer*, vol 50, pp. 1-6.

Roberts, M., Alexander, F., Anderson, T., Forrest, A. P. M., Kirkpatrick, A., Muir, B., et al. (1989); 'The Edinburgh Trial of Screening for Breast Cancer' *The Lancet*.

Professor Jocelyn Chamberlain

At the time of the Forrest Committee Dr Jocelyn Chamberlain was a specialist in community medicine with the South West Thames Regional Health Authority, and Director of the of the DHSS Cancer Screening Evaluation Unit at the Institute of Cancer Research. She is now a part time Professor of Community Medicine at the institute for Cancer Research in London. She is also an ex research fellow (public health) at the London School of Hygiene and Tropical Medicine, and Guy's Hospital, department of Community Medicine.

Relevant publications

Chamberlain, J., (1985); 'Secondary Prevention: Screening for Breast Cancer', *Journal of Epidemiology and Community Health*, vol 38, pp. 54-7.

Chamberlain, J., (1989); 'Breast Screening: A Response to Dr M Roberts', *British Medical Journal*, vol 299, pp. 1336-7.

Chamberlain, J., Clifford, R., E., et al. (1979); 'Error Rates in Screening for Breast Cancer by Clinical Examination and Mammography', *Clinical Oncology*, vol 5, p. 135.

Day, N., Chamberlain, J., (1988); 'Screening for Breast Cancer: Workshop Report', *European Journal of Clinical Oncology*, vol 24, pp. 55-9.

Ellman, R., Chamberlain, J., (1982); 'Psychiatric Morbidity Associated With Screening for Breast Cancer' *British Journal of Cancer*, vol 60, pp. 781-4.

Gravelle, H., Chamberlain, J., (1982); 'Breast Cancer Screening and Health Service Costs' *Journal of Health Economics*, vol 1, pp. 185-207.

Moss, S., Chamberlain, J., et al., (1987); 'Calculation of Sample Size in Trials for Screening for Early Diagnosis of Disease', *International Journal of Epidemiology*, vol 16, pp. 104-7.

Mr Arnold Elton CBE

At the time of the Forrest Committee Mr Elton was an Honourary Consultant Surgeon at Northwick Park Hospital, Middlesex. He has since become a Research Scholar at Charing Cross Hospital. He is an examiner in Surgery of the General Nursing Council, and he is a Fellow of the Royal Society of Medicine.

Relevant publications

Roberts, M., Elton, A., et al., (1986); 'Edinburgh Breast Education Campaign on Breast Cancer and Breast Self Examination: Was It Worthwhile?', *Journal of Epidemiology and Community Medicine*, vol 40, pp. 338-43.

Professor Kenneth Evans

At the time of the Forrest Committee, Professor Evans was Professor of radiology, at the University of Wales College of Medicine. He was (and still is) a member of the British Institute of Radiologists, and until recently was a senior member of the diagnostic radiology team at the Hammersmith Hospital London.

Relevant publications

Furnival, I., Gravelle, H., Evans, K., and Forrest, A. P. M., (1970); 'Accuracy of Screening Methods for the Diagnosis of Breast Disease', *British Medical Journal*, vol 4, pp. 461-3.

Dr Huw Gravelle

Dr Gravelle was a Consultant Radiologist at the University Hospital in Nottingham until March 1986, he then became consultant radiologist at the University Hospital of Wales. He was (and still is) a member of the British Institute of radiologists, and he is also a senior member of the radiodiagnostic department at the Royal Infirmary, Edinburgh.

Relevant publications

Furnival, I., Gravelle, I., H., Evans, K., Forrest, A. P. M., (1970); 'The Accuracy of Screening Methods for the Diagnosis of Breast Disease', *British Medical Journal*, vol 4, pp. 461-3.
Gravelle, I. H., et al., (1986); 'A Prospective Study of Mammographic Parenchymal Patterns and Risk of Breast Cancer', *British Journal of Radiology*, vol 59, no. 701, pp. 487-491.
Gravelle, I. H., Chamberlain, J., (1982); 'Breast Cancer Screening and Health Service Costs', *Journal of Health Economics*, vol 1, pp. 185-207.

Dr Dorothy Hayes

Dr Hayes was a consultant histopathologist at Belfast City Hospital and Honourary Lecturer at the Queen's University of Belfast. She is a part-time member of the Pathological Society of Great Britain and Ireland.

Relevant publications

None.

Professor Charles Joslin

Professor Joslin was professor of Radiotherapy at the University of Leeds. He is a part time member (ex president) of the British Institute of Radiologists, and he is also a member (ex chairman) of the British Cancer Society. HE was also until recently a senior member of the radiotherapy unit at Charing Cross Hospital, London.

Relevant publications

Phillip, J., Joslin, C., et al., (1984); 'Breast Self Examination, Clinical Results From a Population Based Prospective Study', *British Journal of Cancer*, vol 50, pp. 7-12.

Dr Eric Roebuck

From March 1986, Dr Roebuck was a consultant radiologist at the University Hospital in Nottingham, and he is a member of the Royal College of Radiology.

Relevant publications

Dowle, C., Roebuck, E., et al., (1987); 'Primary Results of the Nottingham Breast Self-Examination Programme', *British Journal of Surgery*, vol 74, pp. 217-9.
Roebuck, E., J., (1986); 'Mammography and Screening for Breast Cancer', *British Medical Journal*, vol 292, pp. 223-226.
Roebuck, E., Elston, C., (1989); 'Results From a Seven Year Programme of Breast Self-Examination in 89,010 Women', *British Journal of Cancer*, vol 60, pp. 401-405.

Appendix 3

Table of clinical trials of breast cancer screening

	Number of women invited	Age of invited women	date	screening methods	number screening rounds
Health Insurance Plan	s 30,131 c 30,565	40-65	1963-66	clinical exam +2 view mam.	4
Two Counties (Sweden)	s 77,080 c 55,985	40-74	1977-80	1 view mam.	2
Malmo (Sweden)	s 21,088 c 21,195	40-70	1978-86	2 view mam.	6
Edinburgh	s 23,226 c 21,904	45-64	1978-81	clinical exam +2 view mam.	7
TEDBC (UK)	s 45,088 c 127,117	45-64	1979-81	clinical exam + 1 view mam.	4
BCDDP (US)	283,222 (participants)	35-74	1973-75	clinical exam + 2 view mam.	5
Nijmegen (Netherlands)	19,702 (participants)	35-64	1974-76	1 view mam.	4
Utrecht (Netherlands)	14,796 (participants)	50-64	1974-76	clinical exam + 1 view mam.	3

Appendix 4

Risk factors for breast cancer

Factor	High Risk	Low Risk
Demographic factors		
age	age 50 years or over	age less than 50 years
social class	social class 1 - 3	social class 3 - 5
country of residence	North America and Northern Europe	Africa and Asia
Family History	first degree relative with breast cancer	no close relatives with breast cancer
Previous Medical History	histologically confirmed fibrocystic breast disease	
	previous breast cancer	
	previous ovarian or endometrial cancer	
	early menarche	late menarche
	late menopause	early menopause
	nil parity or first full term pregnancy after age 30	first full term pregnancy before age 20
Other Factors	ionising radiation overweight	ideal weight for height or thinner

Appendix 5

Table of U.K. committees and trials of breast cancer screening

	Forrest Committee	Advisory Committee on Breast cancer	U.K. Trial	B.C.T.C.
Dr J. Cuzick	*			*
Dr E. Roebuck	*	*	*	
Dr M. Roberts	*		*	
A. P. Forrest	*		*	
Dr P. Last	*	*		
Prof. J. Chamberlain	*	*	*	*
B. Roberts	*		*	
A. Joslin	*		*	*
Prof Vessey	*	*	*	
Prof Price	*		*	
G. Harris	*		*	
J. Phillips	*		*	
A. Kirkpatrick	*	*	*	
Prof Baum		*	*	*
Prof. Wald	*	*		
Dr Spittle		*		*
Dr Murray-Sykes	*	*		
Dr S Moss	*	*		
Dr N Day	*	*		
Dr Bourdillion	*	*		
R Ellman	*		*	
S. Moss	*		*	
R. Blamey	*		*	
F. Alexander	*	*	*	*
B. Thomas	*		*	*